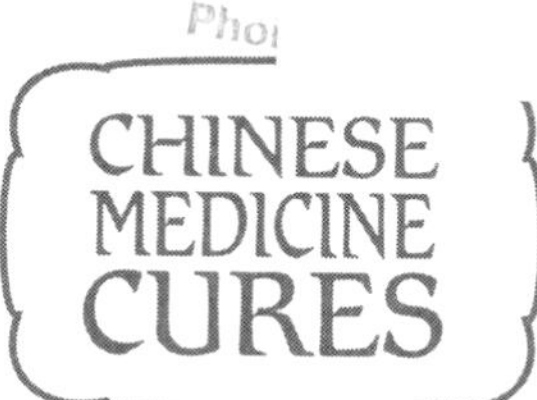

HAY FEVER

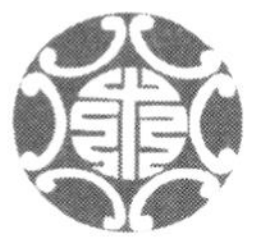

BOB FLAWS

Adapted for the UK by Sylvia Schroer

foulsham
LONDON • NEW YORK • TORONTO • SYDNEY

foulsham
The Publishing House, Bennetts Close,
Cippenham, Berkshire SL1 5AP, England

ISBN 0-572-02576-9

Neither the editors of W. Foulsham and Co. Ltd nor the author nor the publisher take responsibility for any possible consequences from any treatment, procedure, test, exercise, action or application of medication or preparation by any person reading or following the information in this book. The publication of this book does not constitute the practice of medicine, and this book does not attempt to replace your doctor. The author and publisher advise the reader to check with a doctor before administering any medication or undertaking any course of treatment or exercise.

Printed in Great Britain by St. Edmundsbury Press, Bury St. Edmunds, Suffolk

CONTENTS

PREFACE

This is a layperson's book on Chinese medicine and hay fever or allergic rhinitis. The information it contains will also be very helpful for people suffering from allergic asthma. For many years, I myself suffered from both allergic rhinitis and asthma. Since learning Chinese medicine and living by its precepts, I have not had an episode of asthma in many years and do not even own any asthma medication. I do not have hay fever, and I can even be around cats without feeling that dreaded itching in my eyes and constriction in my lungs.

Chinese medicine has helped me to learn what was at the root of my allergies and how to correct my diet, in particular, in order to eliminate my allergies' fundamental causes. As a professional practitioner of Chinese medicine, I have also helped many other Western patients overcome their allergies. Therefore, I know from first-hand experience what Chinese medicine has to offer sufferers of allergic rhinitis and allergic asthma, and my desire to share this valuable information with a larger audience has prompted me to write this book. If you follow the advice it contains, I believe that you too will experience fewer and less severe allergic attacks and that your general level of health and well-being will definitely improve. Good reading and good health!

Bob Flaws

INTRODUCTION

It was spring again and Jim was not happy. For several days, his nose had been running constantly, his eyes and the roof of his mouth itched incessantly, and he couldn't smell a thing. In addition, his eyes were red, he felt frustrated and unattractive, and he was extremely irritable. As a child, Jim had been diagnosed as suffering from seasonal allergic rhinitis. This is the medical name for what most of us call hay fever. Jim had to go to work, a one-hour drive in heavy traffic. Once he got to work, he was supposed to give an important presentation to the board of directors. He had tried over-the-counter antihistamines, but these made him feel drowsy – something he could not afford this morning. What to do?

WHAT IS HAY FEVER?

Hay fever is a group of allergic symptoms characterised by seasonal or perennial sneezing, runny nose, nasal congestion, itching of the eyes, nose and throat, and possible conjunctivitis or red eyes. Usually the itching starts first, followed by the runny nose, sneezing and congestion. Most people are allergic to a range of pollens and find their symptoms worsen at different times during the growing or flowering season. For many people the whole of the summer is blighted by allergic symptoms. Often people who are allergic to one trigger have other allergies. This can sometimes be due to an atopic tendency (atopy is an inherited tendency to develop allergies but not in a specific form). These other triggers include animals, dust mites, particularly their excrement, and fungal spores. Hay fever or allergic rhinitis sufferers may also show other allergic types of diseases such as asthma, atopic dermatitis (eczema), urticaria and hives.

Hay fever affects the upper part of the respiratory tract. Some hay fever sufferers may also develop or suffer from asthma, which involves bronchospasm (spasm of the smooth muscles of the lower airways). The symptoms are breathing difficulties with wheezing and coughing. Hay fever is always an allergic reaction whereas asthma does not have to be triggered by an allergic phenomenon. Whilst some hay fever sufferers also have asthma and some asthmatics have hay fever, the two conditions do not always go together. People may also develop sinusitis, or infection and inflammation of the sinus cavities, secondary to a bout of hay fever. Other symptoms associated with hay fever include frontal headaches (due to sinus congestion), irritability, loss of appetite, depression and insomnia.

WHO GETS HAY FEVER?

Hay fever is an allergy which affects huge numbers of the population. One person in five in the UK suffers from an allergy of some kind and, at a conservative estimate, 17 per cent of the population have allergic rhinitis. One in ten people suffers from hay fever, an estimated nine million people in the UK.

Allergies affect people of all ages, including children. It is believed that there is a genetic component or inherited predisposition involved in atopic allergies. As mentioned earlier, atopic factors may be involved in asthma. Parents and children may both be allergic but not necessarily to the same things. Nearly 25 per cent of children with asthma have more than one allergic symptom, and children who develop asthma when they are older generally have more allergic symptoms.

Apart from genetic factors, it is not known in Western medicine why some people develop allergies and others do not. Some believe that hormonal influences, viral infections, smoking and a number of other factors may affect whether allergies develop or not. We don't really know in the West why people become allergic to different things, or why some have hay fever and others have asthma. There is, however, strong evidence to suggest that allergic diseases are currently on the increase.

WHAT CAUSES HAY FEVER?

People who have allergies are hypersensitive to the things to which they are allergic. When a water-soluble protein molecule of the offending substance enters their system their immune system kicks into action, behaving as if the offending molecule were a cause of disease. The body releases various pharmacologically active substances into the system, such as histamines and other substances that dilate the blood vessels, increase capillary permeability and cause smooth muscle contractions and blood and tissue eosinophilia (an increase in a particular type of white blood cell). In people with hay fever, the offending substances, for example airborne pollens, fungal spores and dust mites, affect the mucous membranes of the nasal cavity and the upper part of the respiratory tract.

Allergic reactions can take place fairly quickly, although they are not as rapid as an anaphylactic reaction, which is very severe and possibly life-threatening. Someone who experiences an allergy may go outside on a bright, sunny day and within 15 minutes start to notice allergic symptoms. Some people also experience late-phase reactions. In this case, the site of the allergic reaction becomes red, swollen, hot and tender, causing a more prolonged reaction. The person may go out at 8 a.m. and experience a late reaction at 4 p.m. Such reactions may also last one or two days, a week or even a month from a single allergen exposure. These kinds of late-phase reactions typically play a part in chronic asthma, rhinitis, eczema and hives.

WHAT ABOUT ALLERGIES TO ANIMALS?

Approximately 10 per cent of the population develop allergic rhinitis when they come in contact with certain animals. For those with asthma, the percentage jumps to 20–30 per cent. Although many people with animal allergies think they are allergic to animal hair, it is the dander – plant and mould allergens clinging to the hair – and proteins within the animal's urine and saliva that are the problem. All animals produce dander and there is no relationship between the length of an animal's hair and its tendency to cause an allergic reaction. While many animals, including dogs, birds, and rabbits, are a primary cause of allergic reactions, the cat is the most allergenic pet.

WHAT ABOUT HOUSE DUST?

House dust is a major cause of allergic rhinitis in people with perennial or year-round symptoms. House dust is a collection of debris from many sources, including fabric fibres, human skin, human and animal dander, bacteria, insect parts, mould spores, food particles and other organic and synthetic materials. While a person may be allergic to any one of these components, the major allergy-causing substance in house dust is a microscopic creature called a dust mite. Mites are members of the same family as spiders. However, dust mites are so tiny they cannot be seen without a microscope. There are 100–500 dust mites in an average gram of house dust. These mites do not bite or otherwise transmit disease, so they pose no health risk except to people who are allergic to them. It is the protein in mites and mite faeces that causes allergies in humans, and the dust mite is now thought to be the most important allergen associated with asthma.

HOW IS ALLERGIC RHINITIS DIAGNOSED?

Usually, allergic rhinitis is diagnosed from its typical recurrent symptoms or, in other words, from the patient's history. This working hypothesis is then confirmed by physical inspection of the mucous membranes and conjunctiva in the eyes. For instance, the conjunctiva are 'injected', i.e. congested and red (bloodshot in layperson's terms), while the mucous membranes within the nose are swollen and bluish red. The role of a particular antigen or offending substance can be determined by skin patch testing. Test solutions are made from extracts of materials that are inhaled or ingested, such as pollens, moulds, house dust, etc. These test solutions are applied to scratches or shallow punctures of the skin. A positive 'weal-and-flare' reaction is usually obvious 7–20 minutes after the extract is applied if a person is allergic to that substance. Diagnosis is also confirmed by the presence of increased eosinophils (a type of white blood cell) in the nasal secretions and by certain antibodies in the blood, although diagnosis by this latter method is expensive.

HOW DOES WESTERN MEDICINE TREAT HAY FEVER?

Antihistamines

The most common Western medical treatment of hay fever is with antihistamines, which were developed about 50 years ago. It is the release of histamines that is responsible for many of the signs and symptoms of hay fever, so antihistamines or histamine blocking agents are used to suppress these symptoms. They are, however, of no benefit to asthma sufferers. An unfortunate side-effect of antihistamines is that they may make you feel dizzy, groggy or drowsy. It is not advisable to operate machinery, or do any work which requires clarity and sharpness of mind, after taking them. The sedative effect of some antihistamines is so marked that they may be given as sedatives to children. Many people are unhappy with the side-effects of antihistamines.

Antihistamines are often available over the counter and do not require a prescription. Common antihistamines in the UK are Telfast, loratidine (sold under the brand name Clarityn), Piriton (a brand name of chlorpheniramine) and Zirtek. Some are now non-sedating and cause less pronounced drowsiness and sedation such as fexofenadine, terfenadine and loratidine. They are, however, more expensive than the more sedating ones, and they may produce more serious side-effects when taken with certain other medications. Antihistamines can aggravate glaucoma, prostatic obstruction and certain kinds of peptic ulcers. They may cause life-threatening ventricular arrhythmias (irregular heartbeat) in people with impaired liver function. Antihistamines also modify the effects of other drugs, such as alcohol and antidepressants.

Decongestants

Sufferers of hay fever often use decongestants. These often contain sympathomimetic drugs, which constrict blood vessels and reduce the thickness of nasal mucosa. They often have just the opposite side-effects of antihistamines, and tend to make people nervous and excitable when taken orally. Nasal decongestant sprays, drops and inhalants are effective for nasal congestion, but do nothing to relieve red, itchy, irritated eyes. In any case, over-the-counter decongestants should not be taken for more than three days at a time, and a person's allergy season may go on for weeks. They are also of limited value as they can give rise to rebound congestion as their effects wear off.

Sympathomimetic drugs and corticosteroids

Sympathomimetic drugs taken orally can raise the blood pressure, produce cardiovascular effects and cause hyperactivity in children. Topical sympathomimetics such as Otrivine should not be used continually for more than seven days as overuse causes rebound congestion. Corticosteroids (synthetic steroids) may also be used to control inflammation. However, if these are used for any length of time, they can have a number of disturbing side-effects. According to Chinese medicine, corticosteroids can actually worsen one of the underlying mechanisms of allergies such as hay fever.

Immunotherapy

If oral allergy medications are poorly tolerated, possibly producing too many side-effects, or if asthma develops, then desensitisation treatment or immunotherapy may be recommended. This consists of injecting an extract of the allergen under the skin in gradually increasing doses. The best results with this type of treatment require year-round injections. The downside of this kind of treatment is that it can provoke massive allergic reactions if the dose is not correct, including hives or urticaria all over the body, asthma and even anaphylactic shock. This therapy must be carried out in a special allergy clinic.

CHINESE MEDICINE AS A SAFE AND EFFECTIVE ALTERNATIVE

As we have seen, the treatment of hay fever and other forms of allergic rhinitis in the West is not entirely satisfactory. Most of the medications have side-effects and none really treats the root of the problem. Traditional Chinese medicine (TCM), however, has a number of treatments for hay fever and other allergies that are free of side-effects when they are prescribed and used properly. Treatment with Chinese medicine can also get to the root of the problem and prevent it from occurring in the future.

Chinese medicine's theory about the causes and mechanisms of allergic rhinitis is empowering in a way in which Western biomedicine typically is not. Knowing that you have a hair-trigger immune system that is hypersensitive to certain pollen molecules, which then provoke the release of histamines and prostaglandins, does not enable you to do much about it except avoid the triggers. The Chinese medical theory about this disease, couched as it is in everyday descriptions taken from the natural world, both enlightens and empowers patients so they can make relevant adjustments to their diet and lifestyle, thereby returning responsibility to individuals for their own health. So now let's turn to a brief introduction to Chinese medical theory in terms of allergic rhinitis.

BASIC CHINESE MEDICAL THEORY AND ALLERGIC RHINITIS

The traditional Chinese medical term for allergic rhinitis is *bi qiu*, 'snivelling nose'. This refers to the runny nose characteristic of allergic rhinitis. The main symptoms of allergic rhinitis – nasal congestion, itchy nose, red eyes and irritated eyes – are all covered in Chinese medicine. Although allergic rhinitis is a modern Western medical disease category, Chinese doctors have been treating people with the symptoms of allergic rhinitis for thousands of years.

THE MAP IS NOT THE TERRAIN

In order to understand and make sense of how Chinese medicine treats allergic rhinitis, you must first understand that Chinese medicine is a system of medical thought and practice distinct and separate from modern Western medicine. This means shifting models of reality when it comes to thinking about Chinese medicine. It has taken the Chinese more than 2,500 years to develop this medical system. Chinese medicine is the oldest continually practised, literate system of medicine in the world. It is best to approach Chinese medicine on its own terms rather than trying to explain it according to Western medical science.

Most people reading this book will probably have some basic knowledge of biology. Whether we recognise it or not, most of us Westerners regard what we learned about the human body at school as the one true description of reality, not just one possible interpretation. If Chinese medicine is to make any sense to Westerners at all, we need to accept that there are potentially other valid descriptions of the human body, its functions, health and disease. In grappling with this fundamentally important issue, it is useful to think about the concepts of a map and the terrain it describes.

If we take the United Kingdom as an example, we can have numerous different maps of this country's land mass. One map might show population. Another might show per capita incomes. Another might show geographical features or simply be a road map. We could also show county boundaries. In fact, there could be an infinite number of different maps of the United Kingdom depending on what you were trying to show and do. As long as the map is based on accurate information and has been created with self-consistent logic, then one map is not necessarily more correct than another. The issue is to use the right map for what you are trying to do. If you wanted to drive from London to Glasgow for example, a road map is probably the best one for the job but is not necessarily a truer or more real description of the United Kingdom than a map showing annual rainfall.

The point I am trying to make is that the map is not the terrain. The Western biological map of the human body is only one potentially useful medical map. It is no more true than the traditional Chinese medical map, and the facts of one map cannot be reduced to the criteria or standards of another unless they share the same logic right from the beginning. As long as the Western medical map is capable of solving a person's disease in a cost-effective, time-efficient manner without side-effects or iatrogenesis (disease or illness caused by treatment), then it is a useful map. Chinese medicine needs to be judged in the same way. The Chinese medical map of health and disease is just as 'real' and every bit as useful as the Western biological map, as long as in using it practitioners and patients are able to solve health problems in a safe and effective way.

In order to understand how Chinese medicine treats allergic rhinitis, we first need to explain some of the fundamental concepts of this medical system. To truly understand the way in which Chinese medicine works, we need to approach it on its own terms. Should you find any of the terms or language used in this book difficult to understand, there is a glossary on pages 141–9 to which you can refer.

At first, the theories and concepts of Chinese medicine may seem a little odd and mystifying. This is because they are so unfamiliar, and not at all what we are used to in the West. The fact of the matter is, however, that Chinese medicine has successfully treated hay fever, allergic rhinitis, asthma and other allergies for over 2,000 years.

YIN AND YANG

To understand Chinese medicine, one must first understand the concepts of 'yin' and 'yang', since these are the most basic concepts in this system. Yin and yang are the cornerstones for understanding, diagnosing and treating the body and mind in Chinese medicine. In a sense, all the other theories and concepts of Chinese medicine are simply an elaboration of yin and yang. Most people have probably already heard of yin and yang, but do not have a clear idea of what these terms mean.

The concepts of yin and yang can be used to describe everything that exists in the universe, including all the parts and functions of the body. Originally, yin referred to the shady side of a hill and yang to the sunny side of the hill. Since sunshine and shade are two interdependent sides of a single reality, these two aspects of the hill are seen as part of a single whole. Other concepts of yin and yang are that night exists only in relation to day, and cold exists only in relation to heat. According to Chinese thought, every single thing that exists in the universe has these two aspects, a yin and a yang. Thus everything has a front and a back, a top and a bottom, a left and a right, and a beginning and an end. However, something is yin or yang only in relation to its paired complement. Nothing is of itself either yin or yang.

It is the concepts of yin and yang that make Chinese medicine a holistic medicine. This is because, based on this unitary and complementary vision of reality, no body part or body function is viewed as separate or isolated from the whole person. The table below shows a partial list of yin and yang pairs as they apply to the body. It is vital to remember that each item listed is either yin or yang only in relation to its complementary partner. Nothing is absolutely or within itself either yin or yang. As we can see, it is possible to describe every aspect of the body in terms of yin and yang.

Yin	Yang
Form	Function
Organs	Bowels
Blood	Qi
Inside	Outside
Front of body	Back of body
Right side	Left side
Lower body	Upper body
Cool, cold	Warm, hot
Stillness	Activity, movement

QI AND BLOOD

Qi (pronounced 'chee') and blood make up the most important complementary pair of yin and yang within the human body. It is said that, in the world, yin and yang are water and fire, but in the human body, yin and yang are blood and qi.

Qi

Qi is yang in relation to blood, which is yin. Qi is often translated as energy and certainly energy is a manifestation of qi. Chinese language scholars would say, however, that qi is larger than any single type of energy described by modern Western science. Paul Unschuld, in my opinion one of the greatest living sinologists, translates the word qi as influences. This conveys the sense that qi is responsible for change and movement. So with regard to Chinese medicine, qi is that which motivates all movement and transformation or change.

In Chinese medicine, qi is defined as having five specific functions:

1. Defence

It is qi that is responsible for protecting the exterior of the body from invasion by external pathogens. This qi, called defensive qi, flows through the exterior or outer part of the body. The defensive qi plays an extremely important role in the development and prevention of allergic rhinitis. As we shall see, when this qi is weak, external pathogens can enter the body, especially in the nose and upper respiratory tract, creating the struggle between the so-called 'evil disease' qi and the body's healthy 'righteous' or 'immune' qi which results in the symptoms of allergic rhinitis.

2. Transformation

Qi transforms substances so that they can be utilised by the body. An example of this function is the transformation of the food we eat into nutrients to nourish the body, which then produces more qi and blood.

3. Warmth

Qi, being relatively yang, is inherently warm and one of the main functions of the qi is to warm the entire body, both inside and out. If this warming function of the qi is weak, then the lack of warmth and resulting cold may cause the flow of qi and blood to become congealed in a similar way to the cold's effect on water – freezing.

4. Restraint

It is qi that holds all the organs and substances in their proper places. All the organs, blood, and fluids need qi to keep them from falling or leaking out of their specific pathways. If this function of qi is weak, then problems such as uterine prolapse, a tendency to bruise easily, urinary incontinence or a runny nose may occur.

5. Transportation

Qi provides the motivating force for all transportation and movement in the body. Every aspect of the body that moves is moved by the qi. The qi moves the blood and body fluids throughout the body. It moves food through the stomach and blood through the vessels.

Blood

In Chinese medicine, blood refers to the red fluid that flows through our vessels as in modern Western medicine, but it also has other different meanings and implications. Fundamentally, blood is the substance that nourishes and moistens all the body tissues. Without blood, body tissues cannot function properly. Additionally, when there is insufficient blood or it is scanty, body tissues become dry and wither.

Qi and blood are closely interrelated. It is said that 'Qi is the commander of the blood, and blood is the mother of qi.'

This means that it is qi that moves the blood, but it is the blood that provides the nourishment and physical foundation for the creation and existence of the qi.

In Chinese medicine, blood provides the following functions for the body:

1. Nourishment

Blood nourishes the body. Along with qi, the blood goes to every part of the body. When the blood is deficient, function decreases and body tissues atrophy (waste) or shrink.

2. Moistening

Blood moistens the body tissues. This includes the skin, eyes, and ligaments and tendons of the body. A deficiency or lack of blood can cause drying out and consequent stiffening or atrophy of various tissues throughout the body.

3. Material foundation for the spirit or mind

In Chinese medicine, the body and mind are considered as one. The blood (yin) supplies the material support and nourishment for the mind (yang), allowing it to become 'bright' (i.e. conscious and productive), and stay rooted in the body. If the blood is deficient, the mind can 'float', causing problems such as insomnia, agitation and unrest.

ESSENCE

Along with qi and blood, essence is one of the three most important constituents of the body. Essence is the most fundamental material the body uses for its growth, maturation and reproduction. There are two forms of this essence. We inherit essence from our parents, and we also produce our own essence from the food and drink we consume and the air we breathe.

The essence that comes from our parents is what determines our basic constitution, strength and vitality. We each have a finite, limited amount of this inherited essence. It is important to protect and conserve it because all bodily functions depend upon it, and when it is exhausted we die. The depletion of essence has serious implications for our overall health and well-being. Fortunately, the essence derived from food and drink helps to bolster and support this inherited essence. So, if we eat well and do not consume more qi and blood than we create each day, then when we sleep at night this surplus qi and, more especially, blood is transformed into essence.

FLUIDS AND HUMOURS

In addition to qi, blood and essence, there are also various fluids and humours in the body. Fluids and humours are a yin–yang pair. Fluids are clear, thin, light and movable, while humours are turbid, thick, heavy and relatively immobile. In Chinese medicine, it is the qi that moves and transforms fluids. If the qi fails to move and transform fluids and humours, these may collect and turn into what is known as 'water dampness'. Since it is qi that moves and transports liquids in the body, it is said that liquids follow the movement of qi.

THE VISCERA AND BOWELS

In Chinese medicine, the internal organs (called viscera so as not to become confused with the Western biological entities of the same name) have a much wider area of function and influence than in Western medicine. Each viscus has distinct responsibilities for maintaining the physical and psychological health of the individual. From a Chinese medical perspective, it is more useful to view each viscus as a sphere of influence or a network that spreads throughout the body, rather than as a distinct and separate physical organ, as described in Western science. It is for this reason that the German sinologist Manfred Porkert refers to the viscera as orbs rather than as organs. In Chinese medicine, the relationship and connections between the various viscera and other parts of the body are facilitated by the channel and network vessel system which I will discuss later.

According to Chinese medicine, there are five main viscera that are relatively yin, and six main bowels that are relatively yang. The five yin viscera are the heart, lungs, liver, spleen and kidneys. The six yang bowels are the stomach, small intestine, large intestine, gall bladder, urinary bladder and a system that Chinese medicine refers to as the triple burner. The functions of the entire body are arranged or described under these eleven organs or spheres of influence. Chinese medicine as a system does not have a pancreas, a pituitary gland or ovaries, as their functions and others are described by the sphere of influence of the five viscera and six bowels. The actual functions of the viscera and bowels are more important and wider-reaching than their physical structure. For example, someone who had had their gall bladder removed would, from the point of view of Chinese medicine, still have the functional aspects of the gall bladder available to them.

Within this system, the five viscera are the most important. These are the organs that in Chinese medicine are responsible for the creation and transformation of qi and blood and the storage of essence. The kidneys, for example, are responsible for the excretion of urine, but in addition they have many other areas of responsibility, or spheres of influence, such as hearing, bone strength, sex, reproduction, maturation and growth, the lower and upper back, and the lower legs in general and the knees in particular.

Visceral correspondences

The Chinese viscera may have the same name and even some functions in common with the organs of modern Western medicine, but they are quite different from them.

Each of the five Chinese medical viscera also has a corresponding tissue, sense and emotion related to it. These are outlined in the table below.

Organ	Tissue	Sense	Spirit	Emotion
Lungs	Skin/body hair	Smell	Corporeal soul	Grief/sadness
Spleen	Flesh	Taste	Thought	Thinking/worry
Kidneys	Bones/head hair	Hearing	Will	Fear
Liver	Sinews	Sight	Ethereal soul	Anger
Heart	Blood vessels	Speech	Spirit	Joy/fright

Each Chinese medical viscus or bowel possesses both a yin and a yang aspect. The yin aspect of a viscus or bowel refers to its substantial nature or tangible form. Furthermore, an organ's yin is responsible for the nurturing, cooling and moistening of that viscus or bowel. The yang aspect of the viscus or bowel represents its functional activities or what it does. An organ's yang aspect is also warming. These two aspects – yin and yang, form and function, cooling and heating – create good health when balanced. If either yin or yang becomes too strong or too weak, the resulting imbalance may lead to disease.

In terms of the cause and prevention of allergic rhinitis, there are four main viscera that are important. These are the lungs, spleen, kidneys and liver. When these four viscera function properly and work together harmoniously, the body does not develop allergies. If these four viscera do not function properly, then the body can develop allergic symptoms.

The lungs

Although the lungs are not actually the root of allergic rhinitis, most people would probably accept that they play a role in allergies affecting the respiratory tract. According to Chinese medicine, the following concepts relating to the lung's sphere of influence may help to explain how allergies are caused and treated.

1. The lungs govern the qi.

In particular, the lungs govern the defensive qi. As was mentioned earlier, the defensive qi defends the body from invasion by external pathogens.

2. The lungs are the delicate viscus.

This means that the lungs are the most susceptible to external invasion of all the viscera. It is also said that the lungs are the 'florid canopy'. This means that the lungs are like a coping stone over the other viscera and bowels. As such, they are also the first organ to be affected by externally invading pathogens 'floating on the wind'.

3. The lungs form mucus.

Mucus is the fluid of the lungs. Lung diseases often involve an abnormality or imbalance of mucus, such as a runny, blocked or dry nose.

4. The lungs govern the bearing down of the qi.

It is the lung qi that moves the qi of the entire body and subsequently the body fluids (which are propelled by the qi) in a downward direction. If the lungs become diseased, the qi then typically flows upwards instead of downwards as it should. This upward flow of lung qi causes sneezing, coughing, chest tightness, and panting and wheezing, or asthma. If the lung qi flows upwards, the body fluids will not descend correctly and may be drafted upwards along with the lung qi, resulting in a runny nose. The connection between the body fluids and the lungs is underscored by a statement in Chinese medicine, which says that the lungs govern the regulation and flow through the waterways.

5. The lungs open into the portals of the nose, while the pharynx and larynx are the doors of the lungs and stomach. This means that lung problems may cause symptoms involving the nose, pharynx and throat. Loss of smell may occur when the lungs are imbalanced or diseased.

6. The lungs depend on nourishment from the spleen.
The source of qi for the lungs comes from the spleen. If the spleen is weak and deficient, then the lung qi, which is dependent on the spleen qi, will also become weak and deficient. Another factor to be taken into consideration is that the lungs and kidneys are said mutually to engender each other. The lungs are the governor of the qi, while the kidneys are the root of qi. This means that the health of the lungs is also dependent on healthy kidneys. If the kidneys are weak and deficient, this will effect the lung qi.

The spleen

The spleen is actually the single most important Chinese organ or viscus in terms of allergic rhinitis. The spleen and its paired bowel, the stomach, are central in the digestive process. The spleen plays a crucial role in the body's ability to transform food and drink into qi and blood. The spleen, kidneys and lungs all play a part in the metabolism and movement of water throughout the body. The role of the spleen is, however, the most crucial with regard to excessive body fluids that gather and collect, transforming into dampness and then into phlegm.

The role of the spleen in Chinese medicine is very wide-reaching and more important than in Western medicine. This is an excellent illustration of how these two systems of medicine differ in their views of the internal organs and their functions. The main functions of the spleen that relate to allergic rhinitis, according to Chinese medicine, are:

1. The spleen governs the transportation and transformation of food and water.

This means that the spleen takes the partially digested food and fluids from the stomach and begins the process of transforming it into qi, blood and essence. A healthy spleen is vital for producing sufficient qi and blood.

2. The spleen governs the qi of the five viscera.

This underscores the crucial role of the spleen as the main source of qi for all the other viscera and bowels.

3. The spleen governs the bearing up of the clear.

The 'clear' in this instance refers to the clear part of foods and liquids. Its opposite is the turbid. If the spleen functions properly, clear qi is borne upwards to empower the sense organs in the head and the higher mental functions. If the spleen is empty and weak, then the clear qi will not rise and the turbid qi will not go downwards. As a result, there will not be a proper production of lung and defensive qi, while dampness and turbidity will collect and transform into phlegm.

4. The spleen is averse to dampness and sweet flavour enters the spleen.

These two statements are important for understanding diet's impact on the spleen and its role in allergic rhinitis. Foods that are either too sweet or too damp damage the spleen and create dampness and phlegm.

The kidneys

In Chinese medicine, the kidneys are considered to be the foundation of our life. Since the developing foetus is shaped like a kidney and because the kidneys are the main viscus for the storage of our inherited essence, the kidneys are referred to as the prenatal root. Keeping the kidney qi strong and kidney yin and yang in relative balance is considered essential to good health and longevity. The most important Chinese medical aspects relating to the kidneys that are relevant in terms of allergic rhinitis are:

1. The kidneys are responsible for human reproduction, development and maturation.

These are the same functions as those described when the essence was discussed. This is because the essence is stored in the kidneys. Health problems relating to reproduction, development and maturation are commonly problems of kidney essence. Excessive sexual activity, drug use or prolonged over-exhaustion can all damage and consume kidney essence. This statement may also be useful in offering an explanation about how a disease may be inherited. It can also give us an explanation as to why people may grow out of a disease as they mature and why that disease may return as they age. In the first case, the disease goes away because of the maturation of the kidney qi, while in the second, it returns because of the decline of the kidney qi with age.

2. The kidneys are the water viscus and the foundation of water metabolism.

The kidneys work in co-ordination with the lungs and spleen to ensure that water is spread properly throughout the body and that excess water is excreted as urine. Problems such as oedema (fluid retention), excessive dryness, excessive day- or night-time urination or even a runny nose can indicate a weakness of kidney function.

3. The kidneys govern opening and closing.
This means that it is the kidney qi that is responsible for the opening and closing of the body's orifices. If the kidney qi becomes weak and insufficient, it may fail to hold body fluids within these 'portals'. The result is that there may be excessive urination, excessive vaginal discharge, chronic diarrhoea or even a chronic runny nose.

4. Kidney yin and yang are the foundation for the yin and yang of all the other organs and bowels and body tissues of the entire body.
This is another way of saying that the kidneys are the foundation of our life. If either kidney yin or yang is lacking or deficient, eventually the yin or yang of the other viscera and bowels will also become deficient.

The liver

The liver is the fourth viscus in Chinese medicine commonly involved in allergic rhinitis. This is because:

1. The liver governs the free flow and spreading of the qi.
Whilst the lungs (and ultimately the spleen) supply the power for the qi to move, it is the liver that allows the qi to move. Movement is an intrinsic quality of qi and movement is necessary for the qi to perform its functions. If the liver loses control over the proper flow of the qi, then, on the one hand, the qi mechanism of the upward movement of the clear and downward movement of the turbid will be affected, whilst on the other hand, qi will become depressed and stagnate, collect and gather.

2. The liver governs upbearing effusion.
Since the qi is considered to be yang, it tends to move upwards, particularly if a lot collects in one place. If the liver loses its ability to control the free flow and spread of qi, the qi typically first backs up and accumulates and then, incorrectly, flows upwards. This may then negatively affect the downward flow of the lung qi and give rise to sneezing, coughing, asthmatic panting and wheezing, headache and red eyes. All of these symptoms may indicate an incorrect upward flow of the qi. It is said that the liver opens into the portals of the eyes. This helps to explain why, according to Chinese medicine, eye problems often involve the liver.

3. Anger is the emotion of the liver and it damages the liver.
The free flow of qi in the body is most easily damaged by emotional causes and, in particular, by anger, stress and frustration. If we are emotionally upset, the flow of the qi in the body is blocked, particularly if we are stressed and tense. This then causes depression and a constraint of the flow of qi that is controlled by the liver. This type of stagnation and constraint of the flow of liver qi due to emotional frustration and stress is called 'liver depression qi stagnation' in Chinese medicine. Conversely, when the liver is out of balance or becomes diseased, there may be signs of anger and irritability.

4. The liver is yin in form but yang in function and liver yang may transform into fire.
This means that the liver has a lot of yang, remembering that qi is yang. If the qi becomes depressed and backs up in the liver, this may easily transform into heat or fire. There are many signs of abnormal heat in the body.

5. Liver fire may invade the lungs.
This illustrates the close relationship between the liver and

the lungs. If depressive heat accumulates in the liver, this can flow into and invade the lungs. It is also possible for lung disease to stir up, aggravate or create further liver heat, especially if there is heat in the lungs.

THE CHANNELS AND NETWORK VESSELS

Each viscus and bowel has a corresponding channel or meridian with which it is connected. In Chinese medicine, the inside of the body is made up of the viscera and bowels. The outside of the body is composed of the sinews, bones, muscles, flesh, skin and hair. It is the channels and network vessels (i.e. smaller connecting vessels) that connect the inside and the outside of the body. It is through these channels and network vessels that the viscera and bowels connect with their corresponding body tissues.

The channel and network vessel system is a unique feature of Chinese medicine. These channels and vessels are different from the circulatory, nervous or lymphatic systems. The earliest reference to these channels and vessels is in *Nei Jing (The Inner Classic)*, a text written around the second or third century BC.

The channels and vessels perform two basic functions. They are the pathways by which the qi and blood circulate through the body and between the organs and tissues. Additionally, as mentioned above, the channels connect the viscera and bowels with the exterior part of the body. This channel and vessel system functions in the body much like an information or communication network. The channels allow the various parts of our body to co-operate and interact to maintain our lives.

This channel and network vessel system is quite complex. There are 12 primary channels, six yin and six yang, each having a specific pathway through the external body and connected with an internal organ (see diagram below). There are also extraordinary vessels, sinew channels, channel divergences, main network vessels and ultimately countless finer and finer network vessels permeating the entire body. All of these form a closed loop or circuit similar to, but distinct from, the Western circulatory system.

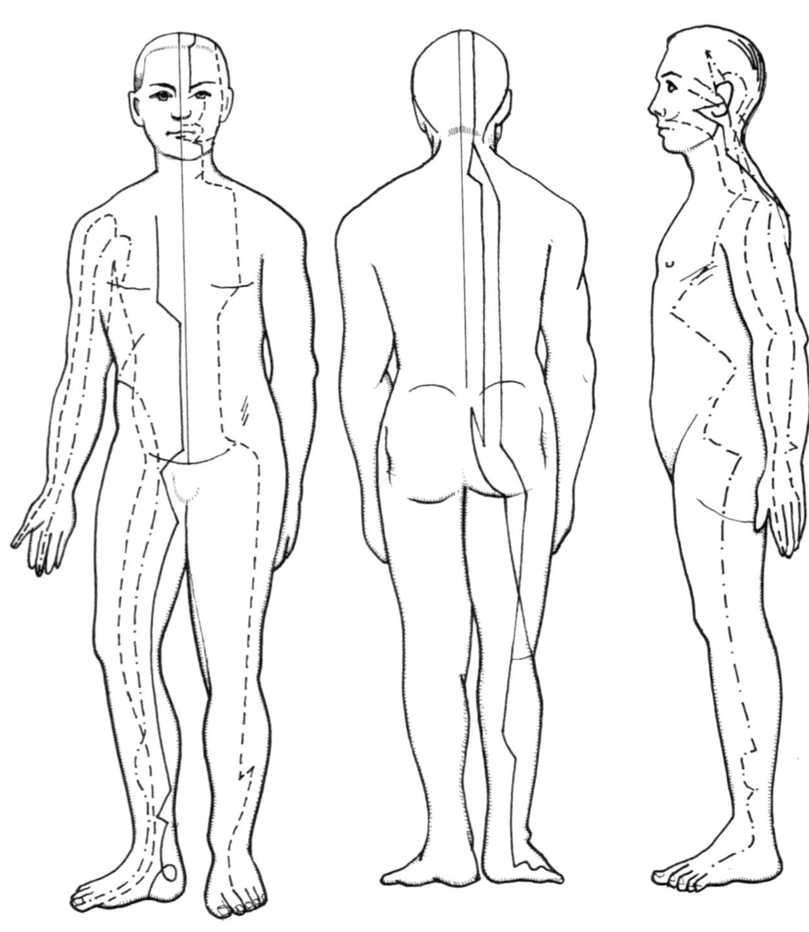

HARMONY AND BALANCE IN CHINESE MEDICINE

Chinese medicine is known as a system of correspondences. In Chinese medicine, nothing stands alone. Every aspect of the body and mind responds and relates to other aspects or functions. The body, mind and spirit form an integrated whole. Health is the harmonious interaction of all the various aspects that comprise the organism. Disease and pain result when there is a disruption to this fundamental harmony and balance. In Chinese medicine, the focus of treatment is therefore on the restoration of harmony.

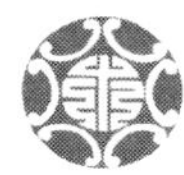

CAUSES OF ALLERGIC RHINITIS FROM A CHINESE MEDICAL PERSPECTIVE

All the signs and symptoms of allergic rhinitis basically involve an imbalance or improper functioning of the lungs, liver, spleen and kidneys. The spleen, as we have already mentioned, is especially important.

INVASION BY WIND EVILS

Let's begin with the actual allergic attack or episode. In Chinese medicine, unseen disease-causing agents, which are in the air around us, are referred to as wind evils. This is similar in concept to the original meaning of malaria – 'bad air'. Chinese doctors in ancient times knew that there was some factor in the environment that precipitated allergic episodes. This factor cannot be seen with the naked eye; it travels through or on the air and it attacks the upper respiratory tract.

If such unseen pathogens or wind evils invade the body, they occupy the space through which the body's normal qi, blood and body fluids flow, thereby displacing them and disturbing the free flow of the body's righteous, healthy qi. With regard to allergic rhinitis, the wind evils enter the body through the mouth and nose. As you may recollect from the preceding chapter, the nose and throat are associated with the lungs. At first, the wind evils cause local congestion in the affected area. Thus one of the first symptoms of the onset of allergic rhinitis is localised itching. This itching is the symptom of a blockage to the free flow of qi and blood in the affected area.

This itching is soon followed by sneezing and a runny nose. As the disease evils of external 'wind' enter the body more deeply, they disturb the function of the first organ they reach. The lungs are the florid canopy or the coping stone of all the other viscera and bowels. They are also a delicate viscus, meaning that they are relatively easily invaded by external evils. The lungs' function is to move the qi down the body. If wind evils disturb this function of the lungs, the lung qi flows upwards instead and results in sneezing. If the lung qi is flowing in the wrong direction, the fluids that follow the flow of the qi may also go in the wrong direction. Fluids may spill over from the portal that is associated with the lungs, so you end up with a runny nose. If lung function is further compromised, you could also end up with coughing and asthma.

Since the lungs and liver are so closely related, if the lung qi flows upwards instead of downwards (as a result of externally invading wind evils), this can also disturb the liver. If there is liver depression qi stagnation (as a result of emotional stress for example) with depressive heat accumulating in the liver, this invasion by wind evils of the lungs may be all that is needed to tip the balance and allow or stimulate this depressive heat to flow upwards to the portal of the liver, i.e. the eyes.

THE PIVOTAL ROLE OF THE SPLEEN

Although acute allergic episodes may be triggered by invasion of the body by external wind evils, not everyone in the same environment will develop allergies. So there must be other factors involved apart from the presence of external wind evils in the environment. *Nei Jing (The Inner Classic),* the so-called bible of Chinese medicine, says, 'If evils assemble somewhere, qi must necessarily be vacuous.' This means that evil qi cannot invade the body of a person whose defensive qi is strong and sufficient, so people who develop allergies have insufficient or weaker defensive qi than others, thus allowing wind evils to penetrate their defences.

The defensive qi is manufactured from food and drink that is taken into the body and transformed by the spleen. The root of defensive qi vacuity or deficiency is mainly spleen qi vacuity. If the spleen qi is strong or fortified, the defensive qi will protect the exterior of the body from attack.

In addition, since the spleen is responsible for the movement of body fluids, if it is weak and vacuous it may fail to perform this function. Fluids may collect and transform into dampness which, if it persists, will congeal into phlegm. Phlegm is produced by the spleen failing to function properly but it actually ends up in the lungs. Hence according to Chinese medicine, 'The spleen is the root of phlegm production, but the lungs are the place where it is stored.' It is phlegm and dampness mainly due to spleen vacuity that form the mucus that runs from the nose. In allergic rhinitis, spleen vacuity is at the root of the defensive qi vacuity that allows for easy penetration of the body's defences. It is also at the root of the phlegm production giving rise to the presence of mucus.

In some people, the spleen may be constitutionally weak and vacuous. In Western culture, spleen vacuity is often endemic due to many other factors connected with lifestyle and diet. All babies start life with an inherently weak spleen since, according to Chinese medical theory, the spleen and stomach do not mature until around six years of age. If the child is overfed or given foods that are difficult to digest, this further damages the spleen and creates a lot of dampness and phlegm. This is why so many babies and young children have allergies and asthma; often a lifetime of allergies is begun by poor feeding practices of new-borns.

Introducing solid foods when the baby is too young means the food is difficult to digest. Some foods are inherently damp or directly damage the spleen. Wheat and dairy products are inherently damp and therefore tend to create phlegm in those with weak digestion, whereas chilled, cold and raw foods, as well as excessively sweet foods, including fruit juices, damage the spleen.

All this means that many children develop allergies not just because their spleens are constitutionally weak but also because of incorrect feeding and diet. Some children will 'grow out' of their allergies as their spleens mature. Other children will not, either because they are constitutionally weak or have been damaged badly by improper diet.

Another reason why the spleen may be vacuous and depleted is because of insufficient exercise, which leads to the creation of dampness and phlegm. The proper functioning of the spleen is very much influenced by obsessive thinking, overwork, worry and anxiety, which all damage the spleen. The emotions of anger and frustration cause liver depression, which then vents itself on to the spleen, indirectly damaging it.

As we have seen, there are multiple factors that can give rise to the spleen vacuity and phlegm dampness that is at the root of most allergic rhinitis: inherited spleen weakness, improper diet, too little exercise and the emotional factors of overwork, worry, anger and frustration. This may explain why people's allergies come and go. One spring, a person's hay fever may be bad and another it is much better even though the pollen counts are relatively similar. Or, for a number of years a person might be horribly allergic to cats and then 'grow out of it' for several years. Then when they are under stress and eat badly, their allergy may flare up again.

THE KIDNEYS' RELATIONSHIP WITH THE SPLEEN

In Chinese medicine, the spleen and kidneys are the two most important organs for proper physiological function and they mutually support and help each other. The kidneys are the 'former heaven' or 'prenatal root'. This means that the kidneys store and are the source of inherited essence. The spleen is the 'latter heaven' or 'postnatal root'. This is because the spleen is the root of creation for both qi and blood, which are transformed from the food and drink we consume each day. The spleen and stomach act like a pot on a stove distilling the finest essence of food and drink into qi and blood, whilst the kidneys provide the ultimate source of heat under the pot. Prenatally, spleen qi is dependent on kidney yang as its root. Spleen qi and kidney yang are mutually interdependent. If one is weak and depleted, it weakens the other.

Defensive qi or defensive yang is a combination of both spleen qi and kidney yang. Hence, inherited tendencies towards being allergic often involve prenatal or congenital kidney vacuity. Since the kidneys do not become fully active and mature until after puberty, kidney vacuity also plays a part in many paediatric allergies. As the kidneys decline with age, allergies, including asthma, may worsen again after the full vigour of middle age. The kidney qi helps the spleen move and transform body fluids: so kidney vacuity may play a part in the accumulation of phlegm dampness. In addition, the kidney qi helps the spleen qi hold the body fluids within the confines of the body. Having a chronic runny nose may be in some part due to kidney vacuity.

THE ROLE OF THE LIVER

We have seen that the liver's job is to keep the qi moving freely and smoothly throughout the body. If the proper functioning of the liver is affected by emotional stress, the flow of the qi is blocked. The qi will become depressed and back up. According to Chinese medicine, in particular a teaching known as five-phase or element theory, when the liver qi becomes stagnant it is most likely to be vented on to the spleen. If this happens, the spleen becomes vacuous and weak.

Another possibility is that the liver qi may flow upwards, assailing the lungs. This upward flow of liver qi aggravates and predisposes the lung qi to flow upwards as well. This means if there is liver depression qi stagnation, the lung qi will easily and readily flow upwards. Allergic rhinitis therefore has a strong connection with a combination of spleen qi vacuity, phlegm dampness and liver depression qi stagnation.

Qi is considered to be yang in nature, and if it stagnates and accumulates, it tends to transform into heat. Heat is also yang and it tends to travel upwards in the body. As we have already mentioned, there is a tendency for liver depression to transform into heat. This is aggravated by the presence of phlegm dampness, which further blocks the free flow of yang qi. This depressive heat may waft up to the eyes, causing them to be red and itchy. It may also drift upwards to the lungs, causing what Chinese medicine calls hot or heat asthma. If it flows up to the nose and sinuses, it may cause sinusitis. If it flows up to the throat, it may cause a sore, itchy throat. If this heat flows outwards into the skin, it may cause hives with raised, red weals. Depressive heat in the liver is also experienced and manifests as easy anger or irritability.

When someone develops hay fever or allergic rhinitis, it can be quite frustrating. No one likes having red, itchy eyes, a scratchy throat, a stuffed, red, runny nose or a constant need to sneeze and blow their nose. This frustration can lead to further liver depression qi stagnation, which, if it didn't play a role in the original creation of the allergic attack, will typically complicate matters once the attack is under way.

ROOT AND BRANCH

In Chinese medicine, there is an important discrimination between root and branch diseases or the root and branches of a disease. Acute allergic reactions are categorised as a branch disease. When such an acute episode occurs, treatment is typically directed at relieving the branch symptoms as quickly as possible. Allergic attacks are precipitated by invasion of wind evils – unseen disease-causing factors that are transmitted through the air or 'on the wind'.

The root of allergic rhinitis and allergic asthma is a combination of spleen qi vacuity with a habitual abundance of phlegm and dampness, plus kidney vacuity and liver depression, and maybe also depressive heat. In my 20 years of clinical experience, this is the pattern I most often see in sufferers of allergic rhinitis and allergic asthma. Some patients will suffer from kidney yin vacuity. Others will suffer from kidney yang vacuity. Some may not suffer from any kidney vacuity at all. Some may typically display more signs and symptoms of liver depression qi stagnation, while others may display less. In women, it is likely the scenario will be further complicated by blood vacuity, due to the role of the spleen in the creation of blood. (This is because women lose blood every month with menstruation.)

Therefore, during the remittent stage between allergic episodes, the treatment of allergic rhinitis and allergic asthma in Chinese medicine is mainly directed at supplementing the spleen and boosting the qi, transforming phlegm and eliminating dampness, supplementing kidney yin and/or yang, and finally supporting the liver to allow the free flow of qi. If there is depressive heat present, this is resolved and cleared in whichever organ (typically the liver and lungs and possibly the spleen and/or stomach) it is lying in.

As we shall see in the following chapters, Chinese medicine has safe and effective treatments, administered both professionally and as home remedies, for both acute allergic episodes and the underlying root of these episodes during the time between attacks. It is my belief, however, that it is the teachings and techniques relevant to treating the root of this condition that are most valuable to Western patients. When short courses of modern Western medicines are used for acute episodes, they often do a satisfactory job with few serious side-effects. If we wish to get to the root of the allergy, however, Chinese medicine is more effective. This means Chinese medicine can help to prevent the recurrence of attacks.

I know this is possible from my own personal experience. As a child, I had horrible hay fever and allergies, which carried on throughout my teenage years and into young adulthood. Often episodes of allergic rhinitis would quickly progress to asthma attacks. My allergies were so bad, I wasn't able to enter a house if there was a cat present. However, since using Chinese medicine, I have not had any problems now for many years.

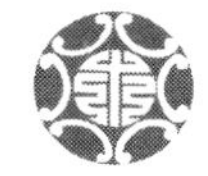

HOW CHINESE MEDICINE TREATS ALLERGIC RHINITIS

TREATMENT BASED ON PATTERN DISCRIMINATION, NOT ON DISEASE

Fundamental to traditional Chinese medicine (TCM) is treatment based on what is known as 'pattern discrimination'. Modern Western medicine bases its treatment on a disease diagnosis. This means that two patients diagnosed as suffering from the same disease will get the same treatment. Whilst TCM does take the patient's disease diagnosis into account, the choice of treatment is not so much based on the disease diagnosis as on what is called the patient's pattern. This aspect of Chinese medicine makes it holistic, safe and effective.

In order to explain the difference between a disease and pattern, let us take the symptom of a headache as an example. All headaches must by definition involve some pain in the head. In modern Western medicine and other medical systems that primarily prescribe on the basis of a disease diagnosis, there is likely to be some sort of specific headache medication given. Headache sufferers can, however, be quite different – man or woman, young or old, overweight or thin, for example. The actual symptoms of the headache can also vary – the location of pain may be left or right side, the type of pain may be throbbing and continuous or sharp but intermittent, etc. One sufferer could also have the following symptoms: indigestion, a tendency to loose stools, cold feet, red eyes, a dry mouth and desire for cold drinks; another sufferer could have a wet, weeping, crusty skin rash with red borders, a tendency towards hay fever, ringing in their ears and dizziness when they stand up. Whilst, according to both Chinese medicine and modern Western medicine, both people suffer from a headache, they also suffer from a whole host of other complaints; they may have very different types of headaches and be of different constitutions, ages and sexes. In Chinese medicine, the patient's pattern is made up from all these other signs and symptoms and further information. The pattern tries to describe the whole person as a unique individual. Treatment is designed to rebalance that entire pattern of imbalance as well as address the major complaint, symptom or disease. There is a saying in Chinese medicine:

> One disease, different treatments
> Different diseases, same treatment

This means that, in Chinese medicine, two patients with the same named disease diagnosis may receive different treatments if their Chinese medical patterns are different; in the same way two patients diagnosed with different named diseases may receive the same treatment if their Chinese medical pattern is the same. The result is that each person is treated individually. There is no allergic rhinitis formula or allergic rhinitis herb. Nor is there any magic allergic rhinitis acupuncture point.

TREATMENT WITHOUT SIDE-EFFECTS

Since every patient receives an individually tailored treatment to restore balance, there are usually no side-effects. Side-effects arise when one part of the body is forced to behave in a way that causes an imbalance in some other part. The treatment may have been appropriate to relieve part of the problem, but it does not take into account the whole. This is a little like robbing Peter to pay Paul. Chinese medicine takes many aspects of a person into account in both diagnosis and treatment and looks at the body and mind as a single, unified whole so that a problem is treated without creating further imbalances.

In professionally practised Chinese medicine, the two main modalities, or methods of treatment, are Chinese herbal medicine and acupuncture. The remainder of this chapter will explore the treatment of allergic rhinitis with Chinese herbal medicine, whilst the next chapter discusses acupuncture.

CHINESE HERBAL MEDICINE

As allergic rhinitis has different disease mechanisms or patterns in different people, it is never treated by a single herb. Chinese herbal medicine is based on rebalancing patterns and these patterns almost always consist of more than a single element. Chinese herbal medicine treatment therefore involves the use of multi-ingredient formulae. Such formulae may have anywhere from six to 18 or more ingredients. If a practitioner of Chinese medicine reads a prescription given by another practitioner, they will be able to tell not only what the patient's pattern discrimination is but also what the likely signs and symptoms are. In creating a herbal formula, the practitioner of Chinese medicine does not just combine several herbs which are reputed to be 'good for allergic rhinitis'. Rather, they carefully craft a formula whose ingredients are designed to rebalance every aspect of the patient's body–mind.

Getting the right herbal medicine treatment

Chinese herbal medicine has become increasingly popular in the West, particularly in the UK. It does, however, require a high level of study as it is quite complex, and it is strongly recommended that you seek professional advice rather than trying to treat yourself. As well as the signs and symptoms of an illness, a practitioner of Chinese medicine will take into account additional information, such as tongue and pulse diagnosis, in order to decide which herbs are appropriate. These skills require experience and training and are beyond the scope of this book. This means that the self-prescribing of Chinese herbs is really not something for the layperson to attempt, especially if unsupervised. As a layperson, it is unlikely that you will be able to obtain Chinese herbs without a prescription from a qualified practitioner in the UK, as reputable suppliers will not generally sell directly to the public. Chinese herbal medicines can be very powerful; just as they have the power to heal, they can also do damage if incorrectly used. Suggestions on how to find a qualified professional Chinese medical practitioner are given on pages 131–4.

In order to demonstrate how a practitioner of Chinese herbal medicine might prescribe a complex, multi-ingredient formula for allergic rhinitis, I would like to present the following textbook description of the Chinese herbal treatment of this condition. This description is taken from *A Practical English–Chinese Library of Traditional Chinese Medicine: Clinic of Traditional Chinese Medicine (II)* (see page 152). The translation is my own.

Internal treatment

Main symptoms

Paroxysmal nasal itching, soreness, distension, sneezing and a great amount of nasal mucus which is clear and watery in consistency, intermittent greyish white nasal obstruction and the possible accompaniment of fatigue, weakness, shortness of breath, disinclination to speak, loss of appetite, loose stools, fear of cold and chilled limbs, back pain, frequent night-time urination, a pale red tongue with thin, white fur and a fine pulse.

Treatment principles

Fortify the spleen and boost the qi, scatter cold and open the portals or orifices (i.e. clear the nostrils of mucus).

Prescription for internal treatment

Bu Zhong Yi Qi Tang (Supplement the Centre and Boost the Qi Decoction) plus *Cang Er Zi San* (Xanthium Powder).

18 g Radix Astragali Membranacei *(Huang Qi)*
9 g Radix Panacis Ginseng *(Ren Shen)*
9 g Radix Angelicae Sinensis *(Dang Gui)*
9 g Fructus Xanthii Sibirici *(Cang Er Zi)*
9 g Flos Magnoliae Liliflorae *(Xin Yi)*
9 g Herba Menthae Haplocalycis *(Bo He)*
9 g Rhizoma Cimicifugae *(Sheng Ma)*
9 g Pericarpium Citri Reticulatae *(Chen Pi)*
9 g Rhizoma Atractylodis Macrocephalae *(Bai Zhu)*
9 g Mix-fried Radix Glycyrrhizae *(Gan Cao)*
9 g Radix Bupleuri *(Chai Hu)*
15 g Radix Angelicae Dahuricae *(Bai Zhi)*

The above quantities make up one day's dosage, to be decocted in water. This formula is for treatment during an acute attack. Then, depending on the individual patient's pattern and symptoms, this basic formula is modified with various additions and subtractions.

If lung qi vacuity is marked, increase the dose of Radix Astragali to 30 g/1 oz and add 9 g Radix Ledebouriellae Divaricatae *(Fang Feng)*.

If there is simultaneous abdominal distension and loose stools, add 15 g/½ oz Semen Dolichoris Lablab *(Bai Bian Dou)*, and 18 g Semen Coicis Lachryma-jobi *(Yi Yi Ren)*.

If there is lower back pain and frequent night-time urination, add 6 g Rhizoma Curculiginis Orchioidis *(Xian Mao)* and 6 g Radix Lateralis Praeparatus Aconiti Carmichaeli *(Fu Zi)* or also administer Jin Gui Shen Qi Wan *(Golden Cabinet Kidney Qi Pills).*

If the soft tissue inside the nose is swollen, add 15 g/½ oz Radix Rubrus Paeoniae Lactiflorae *(Chi Shao),* 9 g Radix Ligustici Wallichii *(Chuan Xiong)* and 9 g Fructus Liquidambaris Taiwaniae *(Lu Lu Tong).*

If the amount of clear nasal mucus is profuse, add 9 g Fructus Schisandrae Chinensis *(Wu Wei Zi),* 9 g Fructus Pruni Mume *(Wu Mei)* and 3 g Herba Asari Cum Radice *(Xi Xin).*

External treatment

1. *Bi Yun San* (Jade Cloud Powder)

30 g Herba Centipedae *(E Bu Shi Cao)*
30 g Radix Ligustici Wallichii *(Chuan Xiong)*
6 g Flos Magnoliae Liliflorae *(Xin Yi Hua)*
6 g Herba Asari Cum Radice *(Xi Xin)*
3 g Pulvis Indigonis *(Qing Dai)*

Grind these into a fine powder and blow into the nose three times a day.

2. *Yu Nao Shi Ruan Gao Pian* (Fish Brain Stone Soft Ointment Tablet)

9 g Powdered Otolith Pseudosciaenae *(Yu Nao Shi)*
0.9 g Borneol *(Bing Pian)*
6 g Flos Magnoliae Liliflorae *(Xin Yi)*
3 g Herba Asari Cum Radice *(Xi Xin)*

Grind into a fine powder and mix with petroleum jelly. Make into a soft ointment tablet and insert into the nose once a day.

3. Massage *Ying Xiang* (LI 20) (an acupuncture point on either side of the wings of the nose) once each day.

The above treatments are given as examples of typical multi-ingredient Chinese herbal formulae for an acute episode of allergic rhinitis. Patients may receive quite different formulae depending on the main characteristics of their individual pattern. The basic formula for internal administration *(Bu Zhong Yi Qi Tang)* is one of the most well-known Chinese herbal formulae for spleen qi vacuity complicated by liver depression qi stagnation. During times of remission where treatment of the root of this condition is required, i.e. spleen vacuity and liver depression, this standard formula is often a very good choice.

Chinese patent medicines

Depending on where you live, the situation with regard to obtaining herbal medicines and your access to a qualified practitioner will vary. In some countries you may be able to obtain a variety of ready-made Chinese formulae in pill and powder form. The remainder of this chapter will look at some of the most widely used patent medicines for the treatment of allergic rhinitis. I would, however, strongly advise you to seek professional advice when taking Chinese herbal medicines.

Cang Er Zi San

This formula is named after its main ingredient, xanthium seeds. It is available as a desiccated, powdered extract under the name Xanthium Formula. Its ingredients include: Fructus Xanthii Sibirici *(Cang Er Zi)*, Flos Magnoliae Liliflorae *(Xin Yi Hua)*, Radix Angelicae Dahuricae *(Bai Zhi)* and Herba Menthae Haplocalycis *(Bo He)*.

All four of these ingredients dispel externally invading 'wind' from the body and specifically open the nasal passageways. This formula is for the symptomatic relief of acute allergic rhinitis. The ingredients in this formula are often added to other formulae that address the underlying root mechanisms of allergic rhinitis, as in the case presented earlier. As this formula only relieves symptoms such as sneezing, nasal congestion and an itchy or runny nose, it is not meant to be taken between attacks. It will not prevent the attacks from coming back again.

Bi Yan Pian

The name of this formula translates as Nose Inflammation Tablets. Like the previous formula, it is primarily for the symptomatic relief of acute allergic rhinitis, and contains the first three of the four ingredients of that formula. It also contains a number of medicinals that clear heat so it is best used if your condition involves heat symptoms. These would manifest as thick, opaque, white nasal mucus, yellow mucus, or even green mucus. Thus, this formula can also be used for acute sinusitis. Like the previous formula, it is not a root treatment, but it can be combined with other formulas which do address the root of the problem.

***Bi Min Gan Wan* (also spelt *Pe Min Kan Wan*)**

The name of these Chinese-made pills translates literally as Nasal Allergy Pills. They are for the relief of acute allergic rhinitis attacks where there is a combination of externally invading wind evils and internally created liver–gall bladder heat flowing upwards. They can also be used to treat acute sinusitis. Their ingredients include:

Fructus Xanthii Sibirici *(Cang Er Zi)*
Herba Agastachis Seu Pogostemi *(Huo Xiang)*
Fel Ursi *(Xiong Dan)*
Calculus Bovis *(Niu Huang)*
Flos Chrysanthemi Indici *(Ye Ju Hua)*
Radix Angelicae Dahuricae *(Bai Zhi)*

Flos Magnoliae Liliflorae *(Xin Yi Hua)*

***Qing Bi Tang* (also spelt *Ching Pi Tang*)**

This is another formula for the treatment of acute episodes of allergic rhinitis and sinusitis. It includes even colder, more powerful ingredients for clearing heat. In this instance, the heat would be in the liver–gall bladder, stomach and intestines and lungs. Other symptoms are a thick yellow or green nasal mucus, constipation, a flushed red face and strong thirst. This formula comes as a powdered, desiccated extract. Its Chinese name means Clear the Nose Decoction. It is sold under the name Pueraria Nasal Combination. Again, this formula is only for the treatment of acute episodes where there is definite inflammation. Its use should, therefore, be discontinued as soon as the attack is brought under control and symptoms of heat have mostly disappeared.

The ingredients in this formula are:

Radix Puerariae *(Ge Gen)*
Radix Ligustici Wallichii *(Chuan Xiong)*
Herba Ephedrae *(Ma Huang)*
Radix Et Rhizoma Rhei *(Da Huang)*
Ramulus Cinnamomi Cassiae *(Gui Zhi)*
Radix Albus Paeoniae Lactiflorae *(Bai Shao)*
Semen Coicis Lachryma-jobi *(Yi Yi Ren)*
Radix Platycodi Grandiflori *(Jie Geng)*
Gypsum Fibrosum *(Shi Gao)*
Flos Magnoliae Liliflorae *(Xin Yi Hua)*
Radix Glycyrrhizae *(Gan Cao)*
Uncooked Rhizoma Zingiberis *(Sheng Jiang)*
Fructus Zizyphi Jujubae *(Da Zao)*

***Xiao Qing Long Tang* (also spelt *Hsaio Ching Lung Tang*)**

The name of this formula means Minor Blue Dragon Decoction. It is available as a powdered, desiccated extract under the name Minor Blue Dragon Combination. It is one of the oldest recorded formulas in Chinese medicine for the treatment of asthma. It can also be used to treat nasal obstruction, sneezing and a runny nose due to allergic rhinitis. Like the preceding formulae, it is meant for the treatment of acute allergic episodes, not for root treatment. Unlike the preceding formula, this one treats cold asthma with copious clear, white, watery phlegm.

Its ingredients are:

Rhizoma Pinelliae Ternatae *(Ban Xia)*
Herba Ephedrae *(Ma Huang)*
Radix Albus Paeoniae Lactiflorae *(Bai Shao)*
Fructus Schisandrae Chinensis *(Wu Wei Zi)*
Ramulus Cinnamomi Cassiae *(Gui Zhi)*
Herba Asari Cum Radice *(Xi Xin)*
Radix Glycyrrhizae *(Gan Cao)*
Uncooked Rhizoma Zingiberis *(Sheng Jiang)*

Su Zi Jiang Qi Tang **(also spelt *Su Tzu Chiang Chi Tang*)**
Su Zi is the name of perilla seeds. *Jiang qi* means to bear down the qi, while *Tang* means soup or decoction. This formula is also for the treatment of allergic rhinitis and allergic asthma. It is used for treating the root condition rather than the branch symptoms. It treats a pattern of phlegm dampness with upward flow of the qi. It can be added to other root formulae described below in order to strengthen their effect of transforming phlegm, eliminating dampness and correcting the flow of qi so it goes downwards. It might be available as a powdered, desiccated extract, sold under the name Perilla Fruit Combination.

Its ingredients are:

Fructus Perillae Frutescentis *(Su Zi)*
Rhizoma Pinelliae Ternatae *(Ban Xia)*

Cortex Magnoliae Officinalis *(Hou Po)*
Radix Peucedani *(Qian Hu)*
Pericarpium Citri Reticulatae *(Chen Pi)*
Radix Angelicae Sinensis *(Dang Gui)*
Ramulus Cinnamomi Cassiae *(Gui Zhi)*
Radix Glycyrrhizae *(Gan Cao)*
Fructus Zizyphi Jujubae *(Da Zao)*
Uncooked Rhizoma Zingiberis *(Sheng Jiang)*

Bu Zhong Yi Qi Tang

Mentioned above under the textbook treatment of allergic rhinitis, the name of this formula translates as Supplement the Centre and Boost the Qi. The centre here refers to the middle burner and the spleen, the most important organ in the middle burner. This is a main formula for supplementing spleen qi vacuity. It also includes ingredients that support the liver and rectify the qi. This formula comes in the form of Chinese and American-made pills, as a tincture and as a desiccated powdered extract sold under the name Ginseng and Astralagus Combination.

The ingredients in this formula are:

Radix Astragali Membranacei *(Huang Qi)*
Radix Panacis Ginseng *(Ren Shen)*
Rhizoma Atractylodis Macrocephalae *(Bai Zhu)*
Mix-fried Radix Glycyrrhizae *(Gan Cao)*
Radix Angelicae Sinensis *(Dang Gui)*
Radix Bupleuri *(Chai Hu)*
Rhizoma Cimicifugae *(Sheng Ma)*
Pericarpium Citri Reticulatae *(Chen Pi)*

***Xiao Yao Wan* (also spelt *Hsiao Yao Wan*)**

Xiao Yao Wan is one of the most commonly prescribed Chinese herbal formulae. Its Chinese name has been translated as Free and Easy Pills, Rambling Pills, Relaxed Wanderer Pills and several other versions giving this same idea of promoting a freer and smoother, more relaxed flow. As a patent medicine, this formula comes as pills and both Chinese-made and American-made versions of this formula may be available. When marketed as a dried, powdered extract, it is sold under the name of Bupleurum and Tang-kuei Formula.

The ingredients in this formula are:

Radix Bupleuri *(Chai Hu)*
Radix Angelicae Sinensis *(Dang Gui)*
Radix Albus Paeoniae Lactiflorae *(Bai Shao)*
Rhizoma Atractylodis Macrocephalae *(Bai Zhu)*
Sclerotium Poriae Cocos *(Fu Ling)*
Mix-fried Radix Glycyrrhizae *(Gan Cao)*
Herba Menthae Haplocalycis *(Bo He)*
Uncooked Rhizoma Zingiberis *(Sheng Jiang)*

This formula treats the pattern of liver depression qi stagnation complicated by blood vacuity and spleen weakness, with possible dampness as well. Although this formula is not for the treatment of acute episodes of allergic rhinitis, it can be used as a root treatment between attacks. Here the liver depression is either more important or equal in importance to spleen vacuity. If spleen vacuity is more important than liver depression, then one of the other formulae below should be used. During acute episodes of allergic rhinitis, this formula can be combined with a patent medicine which targets nasal congestion, runny nose and sneezing more specifically.

Dan Zhi Xiao Yao Wan

Dan Zhi Xiao Yao Wan or Moutan and Gardenia Rambling Pills is a modification of the previous formula, which also comes as a patent medicine in the form of pills. When marketed as a dried, powdered extract, it is sold under the name of Bupleurum and Peony Formula. It is meant to treat the pattern of liver depression transforming into heat with spleen vacuity and possible blood vacuity and/or dampness. The ingredients in this formula are the same as *Xiao Yao Wan* except that two other herbs are added: Cortex Radicis Moutan *(Dan Pi)* and Fructus Gardeniae Jasminoidis *(Shan Zhi Zi)*. These two ingredients clear heat and resolve depression.

Basically, the signs and symptoms of the pattern for which this formula is designed are the same as those for *Xiao Yao Wan* (see page 56), with indications of depressive heat. These might include a reddish tongue with slightly yellow fur, a bowstring and rapid pulse, a bitter taste in the mouth and increased irritability. This formula is also a possible choice for root treatment between attacks when there is liver depression, spleen vacuity and definite depressive heat.

***Xiao Chai Hu Tang* (also spelt *Hsiao Chai Hu Tang*)**

Sold as a powdered, desiccated extract under the name Minor Bupleurum Combination, this is probably the single most frequently prescribed Chinese herbal formula in the world. Like the previous formula, it treats a combination of liver depression, spleen vacuity and depressive heat. It treats depressive heat specifically in the liver, gall bladder, stomach and lungs. It also treats an element of phlegm and not just dampness. It can be used either as a root treatment when there is liver depression, spleen vacuity, heat in the liver, stomach and lungs and phlegm – a very common complicated pattern – or as a branch treatment if combined with one of the other patent medicines described earlier, designed for the first-aid relief of the symptoms of allergic rhinitis, such as *Bi Min Gan Wan*.

The ingredients in this formula are:

Radix Bupleuri *(Chai Hu)*
Radix Scutellariae Baicalensis *(Huang Qin)*
Radix Panacis Ginseng *(Ren Shen)*
Rhizoma Pinelliae Ternatae *(Ban Xia)*
Mix-fried Radix Glycyrrhizae *(Gan Cao)*
Fructus Zizyphi Jujubae *(Da Zao)*
Uncooked Rhizoma Zingiberis *(Sheng Jiang)*

***Gui Pi Wan* (also spelt *Kuei Pi Wan*)**

Gui means to return or restore, *Pi* means the spleen and *Wan* means pills. Therefore, the name of these pills can be translated as Restore the Spleen Pills. When sold as a dried, powdered extract, this formula is called Gingseng and Longan Combination. They not only supplement the spleen qi but also nourish heart blood and calm the heart spirit. This would be the textbook guiding formula for the pattern of heart-spleen dual vacuity. With this pattern there are symptoms of spleen qi vacuity, such as fatigue, poor appetite and cold hands and feet, plus symptoms of heart blood vacuity, such as a pale tongue, heart palpitations and insomnia. This formula is also the standard one for treating heavy or abnormal bleeding due to the spleen not containing and restraining the blood within its vessels. This patent medicine can be combined with *Xiao Yao San* when there is liver depression qi stagnation complicated by heart blood and spleen qi vacuity.

Its ingredients are:

Radix Astragali Membranacei *(Huang Qi)*
Radix Codonopsitis Pilosulae *(Dang Shen)*
Rhizoma Atractylodis Macrocephalae *(Bai Zhu)*
Sclerotium Pararadicis Poriae Cocos *(Fu Shen)*

Mix-fried Radix Glycyrrhizae *(Gan Cao)*
Radix Angelicae Sinensis *(Dang Gui)*
Semen Zizyphi Spinosae *(Suan Zao Ren)*
Arillus Euphoriae Longanae *(Long Yan Rou)*
Radix Polygalae Tenuifoliae *(Yuan Zhi)*
Radix Auklandiae Lappae *(Mu Xiang)*

Again, this formula is meant for root treatment between attacks.

Er Chen Wan

Er Chen Wan means Two Aged (Ingredients) Pills. This is because two of its main ingredients are aged before using. When sold as a dried, powdered extract, this formula is called Citrus and Pinellia Combination. It is used to transform phlegm and eliminate dampness and can be added to just about any formula when there is pronounced phlegm dampness. Its ingredients include:

Rhizoma Pinelliae Ternatae *(Ban Xia)*
Sclerotium Poriae Cocos *(Fu Ling)*
Mix-fried Radix Glycyrrhizae *(Gan Cao)*
Pericarpium Citri Reticulatae *(Chen Pi)*
Uncooked Rhizoma Zingiberis *(Sheng Jiang)*

Assessing over-the-counter medication

If you do try Chinese herbal patent medicines for your hay fever without professional guidance, please be careful. In general, you can tell if any medication or treatment is appropriate for you by checking the following six aspects of your health:

Digestion
Elimination
Energy level
Mood
Appetite
Sleep

If a medication, be it modern Western or traditional Chinese, alleviates your symptoms and these six basic areas of your health also improve, then it is probably a suitable treatment. However, if a treatment or medication causes a deterioration in any of these six mechanisms, even if there is an improvement in your symptoms, then it is probably not the correct treatment and certainly should not be taken on a long-term basis. Chinese medicine aims to rebalance the body's energies and create harmony allowing the body's own natural healing mechanisms to be reinstated. Nothing is more powerful than nature's own healing and this is healing without side-effects.

ACUPUNCTURE

In the previous chapters we have used the traditional Chinese medicine (TCM) point of view to look at the reasons why someone might develop allergic rhinitis and ways of treating it with internal or herbal medicine. This chapter will focus on how Chinese medicine treats hay fever using acupuncture.

Chinese medicine as it has evolved in China has developed in a different social and cultural context from the West and there are differences in how it is practised. In modern China, herbal treatment is very popular. Most Chinese would first think of herbal treatment when considering Chinese medicine and TCM has evolved principally from a herbal tradition. In the West, whilst TCM has played an important role, there have been many other influences. Most Westerners would probably more readily associate Chinese medicine with acupuncture.

Acupuncture has been practised in the UK since the 1960s. It has grown enormously in popularity and there are now many trained practitioners all over the country. We will look at how to find a properly qualified practitioner later on in the book.

Allergic rhinitis and hay fever respond well to acupuncture treatment, although treatment of the root condition may be faster in terms of results with herbal medicine.

WHAT IS ACUPUNCTURE?

Acupuncture involves the insertion of extremely fine needles into specific points on the body. These points lie along the channel and network system described on pages 33–4. By stimulating these points, an acupuncturist may influence the flow of qi or energy in the pathway, thereby influencing the whole energetic system of the person. The aim of acupuncture is to regulate the flow of qi so that there is more balance and harmony in the pathways or channels. This then leads to a restoration of health and well-being.

As we have seen, an acute episode of allergic rhinitis involves a localised congestion of qi and blood and upward flow of the lung and often the liver qi. Since acupuncture's forte is the regulation and rectification of the flow of qi, it is an especially appropriate mode of treatment for allergic symptoms due to qi congestion and an incorrect flow of qi. The insertion of acupuncture needles at various points in the body moves stagnant qi and leads the qi to flow in its proper directions and amounts.

As a generic term, acupuncture also refers to several other methods (apart from the use of needles) to stimulate acupuncture points, thus regulating the flow of qi in the body. One of the other methods is moxibustion (see page 85). This means the warming of acupuncture points, mainly by burning dried, aged Oriental mugwort on, near, or over acupuncture points. The purposes of this warming treatment are: to stimulate the flow of qi and blood even more strongly; to add warmth to areas of the body that are too cold; and to add yang qi to the body to supplement a yang qi deficiency. Some other methods or techniques that may be used by the acupuncturist to stimulate the points are cupping (see page 88), electro-acupuncture and the application of magnets.

WHAT IS A TYPICAL ACUPUNCTURE TREATMENT FOR ALLERGIC RHINITIS?

There are several different styles of acupuncture, so some aspects of treatment will vary from practitioner to practitioner depending on their training, but there are also certain aspects that remain the same. All practitioners will take a case history and gather together information so that they can make a diagnosis. They will almost certainly take the pulse at the wrist[1] and may examine the tongue and palpate the abdomen and the 'channels', looking for areas of tenderness or pain. Once a diagnosis has been made, the practitioner will select points along the channels and will stimulate these points by the use of needles, moxibustion and possibly some of the other stimulation methods mentioned earlier. Nowadays most acupuncturists use disposable needles and are members of professional bodies (see pages 132–4) and as such must comply with strict standards of hygiene and safety.

An acupuncture needle is extremely fine, nothing like a hypodermic needle, and although pain thresholds vary from person to person it is not necessarily a painful therapy. The effect of the treatment may be quite relaxing or even stimulating as the qi is able to flow more freely in the body.

In China, acupuncture treatments are given every day or every other day, three to five times a week, depending on the nature and severity of the condition. In the West, most people visit their practitioner once or twice a week at first and then attend less frequently as their health improves.

In general, it is best to have treatment quite often at first, especially if you are experiencing strong symptoms. Once the symptoms decrease the treatment may be less frequent.

[1] Taking the pulse forms an important part of Chinese medical diagnosis. It is taken from the radial artery at both wrists and there are six different pulse positions at each wrist. These give information about the different viscera, bowels and channels. There are 28 types of pulse quality according to classic Chinese medicine.

HOW ARE THE POINTS SELECTED?

The points where the acupuncturist chooses to insert a needle during treatment are selected on the basis of Chinese medical theory and the known clinical effects of certain points. As mentioned earlier, there are different styles of practice, and point selection may vary from practitioner to practitioner. I will present a fairly typical case here, based on the treatment principles of TCM. This is probably one of the main methods of practising acupuncture, widely used in China, the USA and the UK. It is, however, not the only method so don't worry if your practitioner is not trained in this way or chooses to work in a different way. Diversity of practice is very important in Oriental medicine and enriches the whole field.

Sample case history

The patient's main complaints are itchy eyes and throat, sneezing, runny nose, nasal congestion, fatigue, irritability, chest constriction or stuffiness and slight wheezing. The tongue is very swollen and pale with thin, white fur, so swollen that the indentations of the teeth on the edges of the tongue are clearly visible. The pulse is fine and bowstring. The Chinese pattern discrimination in this example is wind cold invasion disturbing the lungs with upward counterflow, spleen qi vacuity and phlegm dampness. This would be a frequently encountered Chinese pattern of disharmony in young and middle-aged adults during an acute episode of allergic rhinitis.

The treatment principles necessary for remedying this case are to resolve the exterior and dispel wind, fortify the spleen and boost the qi, rectify the qi and move it downwards, transform phlegm and open the portals. In order to accomplish these aims, the practitioner might select the following points:

Ying Xiang (Large intestine 20)
Zan Zhu (Bladder 2)
Lie Que (Lung 7)
He Gu (Large intestine 4)
Tai Chong (Liver 3)
San Yin Jiao (Spleen 6)
Zu San Li (Stomach 36)
Shan Zhong (Conception vessel 17)
Feng Men (Bladder 11)
Fei Shu (Bladder 12)

Ying Xiang, which is next to the wings of the nose, opens the portal of the nose, relieves congestion and stops sneezing and runny nose. *Zan Zhu,* at the inside corners of both eyebrows, relieves the itching of the eyes. *Lie Que* on the lung channel and *He Gu* on the large intestine channel resolve the exterior and dispel wind from the respiratory tract. The combination of *Feng Men* and *Fei Shu,* points on the upper back affecting the lungs, reinforce this action. *Shan Zhong,* on the midline of the chest between the nipples, also helps to regulate and move down the lung qi at the same time as relieving the symptoms of stuffy chest. *Tai Chong,* a point on the liver channel, supports the liver and resolves depression, and also moves and rectifies the qi. It is especially effective when combined, as in this case, with *He Gu.* Together, these two points are very good for calming irritability. *San Yin Jiao,* a point on the inside of the lower legs, is chosen to support the liver further, whilst it also fortifies the spleen. This point is a meeting point for the liver, spleen and kidney channels and is known to promote the nourishment and supplementation of yin blood. *Zu San Li* is a powerful point on the stomach channel. Since the stomach and spleen have a very close relationship according to Chinese medicine, stimulating *Zu San Li* can bolster the spleen as well as the stomach. The stomach channel traverses the chest, and manipulation of a needle at this point can regulate the qi in the chest.

This combination of 10 points addresses the main signs and symptoms according to the Chinese pattern discrimination. It remedies both the underlying disease mechanism and addresses certain key symptoms in a direct and immediate way. This treatment provides both symptomatic relief and, at the same time, starts to correct the underlying mechanisms of these symptoms.

EAR ACUPUNCTURE

Some acupuncturists may also use points in the ear to treat allergic rhinitis. Needles may be used during the acupuncture session or alternatively tiny metal pellets, seeds or special 'press tac' needles, tiny needles which are covered up with tape and left in place for a few days. In this way the effectiveness and duration of treatment may be enhanced.

In terms of allergic rhinitis and asthma, inserting needles at the points *Fei* (Lungs), *Bi* (Nose) and *Ding Chuan* (Stabilising Asthma) can produce beneficial effects by relaxing bronchiole spasm and relieving nasal congestion and a runny nose.

HOW QUICKLY WILL I FEEL THE EFFECTS?

One of the best things about the acupuncture treatment of allergic rhinitis and allergic asthma is that its effects are often immediate. Since many of the mechanisms of allergic rhinitis and asthma have to do with blocked qi, as soon as the qi is made to flow, the symptoms disappear. Many patients can breathe more easily through their nose after the very first treatment. Often people will feel an immediate relief from irritability and tension while still on the table as the qi is flowing more freely. They frequently drop off to sleep for a few minutes while the needles are in place.

THE THREE FREE THERAPIES

All the treatments and therapies we have so far discussed require the aid of a professional practitioner. There are, however, three 'free' therapies that are crucial to treating allergic rhinitis and asthma. These are diet, exercise and deep relaxation. Only you can take care of these three factors in your health!

DIET

In Chinese medicine, the functions of the spleen and stomach are likened to a pot on a stove or a tank in a still. The stomach receives the foods and liquids, which then rot and ripen like a mash in a fermentation vat. The spleen then cooks this mash and drives off (i.e. transforms and moves upwards) the pure part. This pure part collects in the lungs to become the qi and in the heart to become the blood. Chinese medicine characterises this transformation as a process of yang qi transforming yin substance. All the principles of Chinese dietary therapy that may be applied to treat and alleviate hay fever are derived from these basic theories.

We have already seen that the spleen is fundamental to the creation of qi and blood. Based on this concept, a healthy, strong spleen prevents and treats allergic rhinitis in three ways. Firstly, if the spleen is healthy and strong, it will create sufficient defensive qi to protect the exterior of the body from invasion by 'wind evils'. Secondly, since the spleen is in charge of moving and transforming water in the body, a strong, healthy spleen prevents the gathering of phlegm and dampness which could impede the function of the lungs and easily spill over as nasal mucus. Thirdly, the force behind the movement of the qi is mainly derived from the spleen qi which then empowers the lungs. Therefore, if there is sufficient healthy spleen qi, there is a good 'push' behind the movement of qi. This push helps counterbalance or control any tendency of the liver to constrict or constrain the qi flow. According to Chinese medicine, a healthy spleen helps regulate the liver and keep it free from depression and stagnation.

With regards to Chinese dietary therapy and respiratory allergies, the two main issues are to avoid foods that (1) damage the spleen and (2) create dampness and, therefore, phlegm.

Foods that damage the spleen

In terms of foods that damage the spleen we begin with uncooked and especially chilled foods. In Chinese medicine the process of digestion is likened to cooking, which is seen as a type of predigestion before the food enters the body. It is therefore desirable that the overwhelming majority of all food should be predigested, i.e. cooked. Although cooking may destroy some vital nutrients (including qi), cooking does render the remaining nutrients so they are more easily assimilated. This means that even though some nutrients have been lost, the net absorption of nutrients is greater with cooked foods than raw. Furthermore, eating raw foods makes the spleen work harder and can overtax it. If the spleen is very robust, eating uncooked, raw foods may not be too damaging, but it has been shown that the allergic patients' spleen is already weak. It is also a fact that the spleen is constitutionally weak in youngsters and inevitably weakens again with age.

Chilled foods even more than raw foods may directly damage the spleen. Chilled or frozen foods and drinks neutralise the spleen's yang qi. The process of digestion involves warming and digesting all food and drink to 100°F within the stomach so that it may undergo 'distillation'. If the spleen expends too much yang qi just warming the food up, then it will become damaged and weak. So food and drink should be consumed at room temperature at the least and preferably at body temperature. The more signs and symptoms of spleen vacuity or deficiency that a person presents, such as fatigue, chronically loose stools, undigested food in the stools, cold hands and feet, dizziness on standing up and aversion to cold, the more they need to avoid uncooked, chilled foods and drinks.

Additionally, an excess of sugars and sweet things directly damages the spleen. They are inherently dampening according to Chinese medicine. This is because the body creates or secretes fluids that gather and collect, transforming into dampness, in response to an excess of sweet food and drink. The spleen is averse to dampness. Dampness is a yin substance and controls or checks yang qi, which is very important to the proper functioning of the spleen. So anything that is excessively dampening damages the spleen. The sweeter a food is, the more dampening and, therefore, more damaging it is to the spleen.

Foods that create dampness and phlegm

Other foods that are dampening and therefore damaging to the spleen are known as 'sodden wheat foods'. This means flour products such as bread and noodles. Wheat (as opposed to rice) is damp by nature. When wheat is steamed, yeasted and/or refined, it becomes even more dampening. In addition, all oils and fats are damp by nature and may damage the spleen. The more oily or greasy a food is, the worse it is for the spleen. Since milk contains a lot of fat, dairy products are another spleen-damaging, dampness-producing food. This includes milk, butter and cheese.

If we add all this up, then ice cream is just about the worst thing a person with a weak, damp spleen could eat. Ice cream is chilled, it is intensely sweet and it is filled with fat. So it is a triple whammy when it comes to damaging the spleen. In the same way, pasta smothered in tomato sauce and cheese is a recipe for disaster. Pasta made from wheat flour is dampening, tomatoes are dampening and cheese is dampening. Most people don't realise that a glass of fruit juice may contain as much sugar as a sweet bar; fruit juice is also very damaging to the spleen and produces damp.

Below is a list of specific Western foods which, because they are either uncooked, chilled, too sweet, or too dampening, are damaging to the spleen. People with respiratory allergies should avoid these, or minimise their consumption in proportion to how weak and damp their spleen is.

Ice cream
Sugar
Sweets, especially chocolate
Milk
Butter
Cheese
Yoghurt
Raw salads
Fruit juices
Juicy, sweet fruits, such as oranges, peaches, strawberries and tomatoes
Fatty meats
Fried foods
Refined flour products
Cakes and biscuits
Yeasted bread
Nuts
Alcohol (which is essentially sugar)

If the spleen is weak and wet, it is best not to eat too much of anything at any one time. A weak spleen can be overwhelmed by a large meal, especially if any of the food is hard to digest. This then results in food stagnation which impedes the free flow of qi all the more and causes further damage to the spleen.

A clear, bland diet

In Chinese medicine, the best diet for the spleen and therefore, by extension, for most humans, is what is called a 'clear, bland diet'. This is a diet high in complex carbohydrates such as unrefined grains, especially rice and beans. It is also high in lightly cooked vegetables and low in fatty meats, oily, greasy, fried foods and very sweet foods. However, it is not a completely vegetarian diet. Most people, in my experience, should eat 25–50 g/1–2 oz of meat two to four times per week. This animal flesh could be chicken and fish, but should also include some lean beef, pork and lamb. Some fresh or cooked fruits may be eaten, but fruit juices should be avoided. Women especially should make an effort to include tofu and tempeh in their diet, two soya foods now commonly available in health food shops and good supermarkets.

If the spleen is weak, then it is best to eat smaller, more frequent meals. Rice is an excellent food too for three reasons. Firstly, it is neutral in temperature; secondly it fortifies the spleen thereby supplementing the qi; and thirdly, it eliminates dampness. Rice should be the staple grain in the diet.

A few problem foods

There are a few 'problem' foods which deserve special mention.

Coffee

There are two reasons why many people crave coffee. Firstly, coffee moves stuck qi. So, if a person suffers from liver depression qi stagnation, temporarily coffee will make them feel that their qi is flowing. Secondly, coffee transforms essence into qi and makes that qi temporarily available to the body. This means that people who suffer from spleen and/or kidney vacuity fatigue will get a temporary lift from coffee. It will make them feel as if they have energy. However, once this energy is used up, they are left with a negative deficit. The coffee has transformed some of the essence stored in the kidneys into qi. This qi has been used and now there is less stored essence. Since the blood and essence share a common source, coffee drinking may ultimately worsen depression associated with blood or kidney vacuities. Tea has a similar effect as it transforms yin essence into yang qi but the quantity of caffeine in black tea is usually only half that found in coffee.

Chocolate

Chocolate is a combination of oil, sugar and cocoa. We have seen that both oil and sugar are dampening and damaging to the spleen. Temporarily, the sugar will boost the spleen qi, but ultimately it will result in 'sugar blues' or a hypoglycaemic let-down. Cocoa stirs the life gate fire, another name for kidney yang or kidney fire, which is the source of sexual energy and desire. It is said that chocolate is the food of love and from the Chinese medical point of view, that is true. Since chocolate stimulates kidney fire at the same time as it temporarily boosts the spleen, it does give one a rush of yang qi. This rush of yang qi does move depression and stagnation, at least in the short-term. So it makes sense that some people with liver depression, spleen vacuity and kidney yang debility might crave chocolate.

Alcohol

Alcohol is both damp and hot according to Chinese medical theory. It strongly moves the qi and blood. So people with liver depression qi stagnation will feel temporarily better from drinking alcohol. The sugar in alcohol damages the spleen and creates dampness which 'gums up the works' whilst the heat (yang) in alcohol can waste the blood (yin) and aggravate or inflame depressive liver heat.

Hot, peppery foods

Spicy, peppery, 'hot' foods also move the qi, thereby giving some temporary relief to liver depression qi stagnation. However, like alcohol, the heat in hot, spicy foods wastes the blood and can inflame yang. People who run cold and damp can and should eat some hot, peppery foods. However, people with signs of heat congestion, such as thick, yellow mucus, whether from the lungs or sinuses, should steer clear of hot, peppery foods.

Sour foods

In Chinese medicine, the sour flavour is inherently astringent and constricting. People with liver depression qi stagnation should be careful not to use vinegar and other intensely sour foods. Such sour-flavoured foods will only aggravate the qi stagnation by constricting body tissues and further restricting the qi and blood. This is also why sweet and sour foods, such as orange juice and tomatoes, are particularly bad for people with liver depression and spleen vacuity. The sour flavour constricts the qi, while the sweet flavour damages the spleen and creates dampness.

Diet drinks

In my experience, diet drinks containing artificial sweeteners seem to contain something that damages the Chinese concept of the kidneys. I say this because a number of my patients over the years have reported that, when they drink a lot of diet drinks, they experience urinary incontinence and low back and knee pain and weakness. If they stop, these symptoms disappear. Taken as a group, according to Chinese medicine, these are kidney vacuity symptoms. Since many sufferers of respiratory allergies and especially chronic asthma tend to have concomitant kidney vacuity, I recommend patients to steer clear of diet drinks so as not to weaken the kidneys any further or faster.

Some last words on diet

In conclusion, Western patients are always asking me what they should eat in order to cure their disease. Unfortunately, when it comes to diet, the issue is not so much what to eat as what not to eat. Diet most definitely plays a major role in the cause and perpetuation of many people's respiratory allergies, but, except in the case of vegetarians suffering from blood or yin vacuities, the issue is mainly what to avoid or minimise, not what to add. Most of us know that coffee, chocolate, sugars and sweets, oils and fats and alcohol are not good for us. Most of us know that we should be eating more complex carbohydrates and freshly cooked vegetables and less fatty meats. However, it's one thing to know these things and another to follow what we know.

To be perfectly honest, a clear, bland diet as recommended according to the principles of Chinese medicine is not the most exciting diet in the world. It is, however, quite a traditional type of diet and many of our great-grandparents would have eaten like this. Our modern Western diet, which is high in oils and fats, high in sugars and sweets, high in animal proteins and proportionally high in uncooked, chilled foods and drinks, is a relatively recent phenomenon and you can't fool Mother Nature.

When you change to the clear, bland diet of Chinese medicine, you might find that at first you suffer from cravings for more tasty food. These cravings are, in many cases, actually associated with food 'allergies'. We may crave what is actually not good for us just as an alcoholic craves alcohol. After a few days, these cravings tend to disappear and you will find that you don't miss some of the convenience or 'comfort' foods as much as you thought you would. Perseverance is the key to long-term success. As the Chinese say, a million is made up of nothing but lots of ones and a bucket is quickly filled by steady drips and drops.

EXERCISE

Exercise is the second of what I call the three 'free' therapies. According to Chinese medicine, regular and adequate exercise has three basic benefits for sufferers of respiratory allergies. Firstly, exercise promotes the movement of the qi and quickening of the blood. Most respiratory allergies involve an upward qi counterflow caused or at least aggravated by qi stagnation. Exercise can help resolve this, it benefits the liver and corrects the flow of qi.

Secondly, exercise benefits the spleen. The spleen's movement and transportation of digested food is dependent upon the qi mechanism. The qi mechanism describes the function of the qi in moving up and down the pure and turbid parts of digestion respectively. For the qi mechanism to function properly, the qi must be flowing normally and freely. Since exercise moves and rectifies the qi, it also helps regulate and rectify the qi mechanism. The result is that the spleen is able to function well, creating and transforming qi and blood.

If the spleen qi is healthy and strong, the defensive qi will be strong and will protect the body from external invasion by wind evils. In addition, a strong, healthy spleen is capable of moving and transforming water in the body. Allergic rhinitis and asthma both involve phlegm and fluids collecting in the lungs, impeding their function and potentially overflowing. So ensuring that the spleen is strong and healthy prevents the accumulation of dampness and phlegm.

Adequate exercise therefore is a vitally important component to someone suffering with allergic rhinitis.

Aerobics

In my experience, I find aerobic exercise to be the most beneficial for the majority of people with respiratory allergies. By aerobic exercise, I mean any physical activity that raises the heartbeat 80 per cent above normal resting rate and keeps it there for at least 20 minutes. To calculate your normal resting heart rate, place your fingers over the pulsing artery on the front side of your neck. Count the beats for 15 seconds and then multiply by four. This gives you your beats per minute, or BPM. Now multiply your BPM by 0.8. Take the resulting number and add it to your resting BPM. This gives you your aerobic threshold of BPM. Next engage in any physical activity you like. After you have been exercising for five minutes, take your pulse for 15 seconds once again at the artery on the front side of your throat. Again multiply the resulting count by four and this tells you your current BPM. If this number is less than your aerobic threshold BPM, then you know you need to exercise harder or faster. Once you get your heart rate up to your aerobic threshold, then you need to keep exercising at the same level of intensity for at least 20 minutes. Take your pulse every five minutes or so to ensure your heartbeat is being kept high enough.

Depending on your age and physical condition, you will require different types of exercise to reach your aerobic threshold. For some people, simply walking briskly will raise their heartbeat 80 per cent above its resting rate. Others will need to do callisthenics, running, swimming, squash, or some other more strenuous exercise. It really does not matter what the exercise is as long as it raises your heartbeat 80 per cent above its resting rate and keeps it there for 20 minutes. My advice is that you go for something you enjoy and don't find too boring, otherwise you won't want to keep it up. You should also try to make sure that it doesn't cause you any problems or damage to any parts of the body. For example, running on pavements may cause knee problems for some people.

When doing aerobic exercise, it is best to exercise either every day or every other day. If you do not do your aerobics at least once every 72 hours, then its cumulative effects won't be as good. I recommend that my patients with hay fever do some sort of aerobic exercises every day or every other day, three to four times per week at least. The good news is that there is no real need to exercise more than 30 minutes at any one time. A session of 45 minutes is not going to be all that much better than one of 25 minutes, and 25 minutes four times per week is very much better than one hour once a week.

Exercise-induced asthma

Although exercise does not bring on episodes of allergic rhinitis, exercise can induce asthma attacks in some people, so take care if you suffer from asthma. My advice would be to start exercising gently. In the meantime, really sort out your diet. Avoid foods which damage the spleen and foods which produce dampness and phlegm. As your signs and symptoms associated with spleen and kidney vacuity or with phlegm dampness begin to disappear, gradually introduce more strenuous exercise.

DEEP RELAXATION

As we have seen, allergic rhinitis and asthma are commonly associated with liver depression qi stagnation. Even though this may not be the pivotal disease mechanism, it is usually a major contributory mechanism. If liver depression endures or is severe, it typically transforms into heat or fire. Heat and fire, being yang, tend to waft upwards, collecting in the canopy above, the lungs. This heat may be hidden most of the time, but becomes apparent when some other factor pushes it over the edge. According to Chinese medicine, heat from a depressed liver not only tends to collect in the lungs, it is also transmitted to the stomach and gall bladder. The stomach and gall bladder channels both traverse the head over and around the location of the sinuses. Therefore, sinusitis usually involves heat in the liver and lungs as well as the stomach and gall bladder channels.

Liver depression comes from emotional upset and frustration. To an extent these are part of life and we will all have a certain amount of liver depression. When we suffer emotional upset and frustration, our qi becomes depressed. We will feel irritable and tense. When qi becomes depressed in the liver, it accumulates like hot air in a balloon. Eventually, that hot, depressed, angry qi has to go somewhere and it moves upwards in the body.

Essentially, this type of anger and irritability are due to a maladaptive coping response that is typically learned at a young age. When we feel frustrated, stressed or angry about something, most of us tense our muscles, especially the muscles in our upper back and shoulders, neck and jaws. At the same time, many of us will hold our breath. In Chinese medicine, the sinews are governed by the liver. This tensing of the muscles, i.e. the sinews, constricts the flow of qi in the channels and network vessels. Since it is the liver that is responsible for the allowing the movement of qi, such tensing of the sinews leads to liver depression qi stagnation. Since the lungs govern the downward spreading and movement of the qi, holding our breath due to stress or frustration only worsens this tendency of the qi to remain immobile and, therefore, to become depressed in the Chinese medical idea of the liver.

Deep relaxation, therefore, is the third of the three 'free' therapies. For deep relaxation to be therapeutic medically, it needs to bring more than just mental equilibrium. It needs to involve bodily relaxation as well as mental repose. According to Chinese medicine, every emotion is associated with a change in the direction or flow of qi. As I have already said, anger makes the qi move upwards. Fear, on the other hand, makes the qi move downwards. All thoughts and emotions are not just mental but also bodily events. This is why it is not just enough to clear your mind. Clearing your mind is good, but for really marked therapeutic results, it is even better if you clear your mind at the same time as relaxing every muscle in your body as well as your breath.

GUIDED DEEP RELAXATION TAPES

An effective way to practise such mental and physical deep relaxation is to undertake a daily, guided, progressive, deep relaxation session with the aid of an audiotape. It is guided in the sense that a narrator on the tape leads you through the process of deep relaxation. These tapes normally lead you to relax your body in a progressive manner, first relaxing one part and then moving on to another.

There are many such tapes available, and they are often sold in health food shops. Choose several tapes and that way you won't get too bored of listening to the same one. When looking for a good relaxation tape, firstly ensure that the tape is a guided tape and not a subliminal relaxation tape. Subliminal tapes usually have music and any instructions to relax are given so quietly that they are not consciously heard. Although such tapes can help you feel relaxed when you use them, ultimately they do not teach you how to relax as a skill which you can then consciously practise. Secondly, make sure the narrative starts from the top of the body and works downwards. This is because anger makes the qi go upwards in the body, and frustration and anger due to liver depression qi stagnation mean there is already too much qi rising upwards in the body. This depressed qi needs not only to be moved but also to be moved downwards. Thirdly, make sure the tape instructs you to relax your physical body. If you do not relax all your muscles or sinews, the qi cannot flow freely and the liver cannot be coursed. The tape will not be so beneficial if you don't relax your muscles. Finally, try to make sure that the tape instructs you to let your breath go with each exhalation. One of the symptoms of liver depression is a stuffy feeling in the chest which we then subconsciously try to relieve by sighing. Letting each exhalation go completely helps the lungs push the qi downwards.

The importance of daily practice

I was once taken on a field trip to a hospital clinic where they were using deep relaxation as a therapy with patients suffering from high blood pressure, heart disease, strokes, migraines and insomnia. The doctors at this clinic showed me various graphs plotting their research data on how such daily, progressive, deep relaxation can regulate the blood pressure and body temperature and improve the appetite, digestion, elimination, sleep, energy and mood. One of the things they said has stuck with me for 15 years: 'Small results in 100 days, big results in 1,000.' This means that if one does such daily, progressive, deep relaxation every single day for 100 days, certain results will definitely be experienced. What are these 'small' results? Improvements in all the parameters listed above: blood pressure, body temperature, appetite, digestion, elimination, sleep, energy and mood. The 'big' results experienced in 1,000 days of practice are more fundamental.

They really are about a change in how one reacts to stress and are much more permanent.

What these doctors in Shanghai stressed, and what I have also experienced both personally and with my patients, is that the effects of this relaxation are cumulative, meaning that the longer this routine can be practised on a consistent daily basis, the greater and more lasting the effects will be.

It is vitally important to do such guided, progressive, deep relaxation on a daily basis for at the very least three months and ideally for three years. If you achieve this goal, then you will see every parameter of health and well-being improve. If you do this kind of deep relaxation sporadically, missing a day here and there, it will have some benefit, but it will not have the marked, cumulative therapeutic effects that are possible.

The real test

Doing a daily deep relaxation regime is only practice. It's like hitting tennis balls against a wall or hitting a bucket of balls at a driving range: it's not the real thing. The real purpose of a daily deep relaxation regime is not just to relieve the immediate stress and strain but also to learn a new skill, a new way to react to stress. The ultimate goal is to recondition how you react in stressful situations, learning how to breathe out and relax your muscles rather than holding your breath and tensing your muscles. This is the real test, the game of life. Remember: 'Small results in 100 days, big results in 1,000.'

FINDING THE TIME

If you're like me and most of my patients, you are probably asking yourself right now, 'This is all well and good, but when am I supposed to find the time to eat well-balanced cooked meals, exercise at least every other day and do a deep relaxation every day? I'm already stretched to breaking point.' I know. That's the problem.

As a clinician, I often wish I could wave a magic wand over my patients' heads and make them all healthy and well. I cannot. After close to two decades of working with thousands of patients, I know of no easy way to health. There is good living and there is easy living. Or perhaps I am saying this all wrong. What most people take as the easy way these days is to continue pushing their limits to the maximum. The so-called path of least resistance will actually lead to much bigger problems. Unless you take time for yourself and find the time to eat well, exercise and relax, no treatment is going to eliminate your allergies completely. There is simply no pill you can pop or food you can eat that will get rid of the root causes of allergic diseases: poor diet, too little exercise and too much stress.

Even Chinese herbal medicine and acupuncture can only get their full effect if the diet and lifestyle is first adjusted. Sun Si-maio, the most famous Chinese doctor of the Tang dynasty (618–907 AD), who himself refused government office and lived to be 101, said, 'First adjust the diet and lifestyle and only secondarily give herbs and acupuncture.' Likewise, it is said today in China, 'Three parts treatment, seven parts nursing.' This means that any cure is only 30 per cent due to medical treatment and 70 per cent due to nursing, i.e. proper diet and lifestyle.

In my experience, this is absolutely true. Seventy per cent of all disease will improve after three months of proper diet, exercise, relaxation and lifestyle modification. Seventy per cent! Each of us has certain nondiscretionary rituals we perform each day. For instance, you may always and without exception find the time to brush your teeth or shower. The same applies to good eating, exercise and deep relaxation. Where there's a will there's a way. If your allergies are bad enough, you can find the time to eat well, get proper exercise and do a daily deep relaxation tape.

THE SOLUTION TO ALLERGIES IS IN YOUR HANDS

In Boulder, Colorado, where I live, we have a pedestrian precinct in the centre of town. On summer evenings, my wife and I often walk down this mall. Having treated so many people over the years, it is not unusual for me to meet former patients on these strolls. Frequently when we say hello, these patients begin by telling me they are sorry they haven't been in to see me in such a long time. They usually say this apologetically as if they have done something wrong! When I ask if they've been all right they often tell me, 'When my symptoms flare up, I remember what you told me about my diet, exercise and lifestyle. I then go back to doing my exercise or deep relaxation or I change my diet and my symptoms go away. That's why I haven't been in. I'm sorry.'

These patients have no need to apologise. This kind of story is music to my ears. When I hear that these patients are now able to control their own conditions by following the dietary and lifestyle advice I gave them, I know that, as a Chinese doctor, I have done my job correctly. In Chinese medicine, the inferior doctor treats disease after it has appeared. The superior doctor prevents disease before it has arisen. If I can teach my patients how to cure their symptoms themselves by making changes in their diet and lifestyle, then I'm approaching the goal of the high-class Chinese doctor – the prevention of disease through patient education.

The professional practice of medicine is a strange business. We doctors are, or at least should be, always engaged in putting ourselves out of business. Therefore, patients have no need to apologise to me when they tell me they now have control over their health and disease in their own hands.

To achieve these benefits, you must make the necessary changes in eating and behaviour. In addition, allergies and asthma are not conditions that are cured once and for ever like measles or mumps. When I say Chinese medicine can cure allergic rhinitis and asthma, I do not mean that you will never experience a runny nose or chest oppression again. What I mean is that Chinese medicine can eliminate or greatly reduce your symptoms as long as you keep your diet and lifestyle together. People being people, we all 'fall off the wagon' from time to time and we all 'choose our own poisons'. I do not expect perfection from either my patients or myself. I try to give my patients an understanding of what causes their disease and what they can do to minimise or eliminate its causes and mechanisms. It is then up to them to decide what is bearable and what is unbearable or what is an acceptable level of health. The Chinese doctor will have done his or her job when you know how to correct your health to the level you find acceptable, given the price you have to pay.

SIMPLE HOME REMEDIES FOR HAY FEVER

An incorrect diet, lack of adequate exercise and too much stress are the ultimate causes of most allergies, according to Chinese medicine. So making these lifestyle changes is fundamental to the treatment and prevention of allergic rhinitis and asthma. This chapter will focus on a number of simple Chinese home remedies to help relieve the symptoms of respiratory allergies and improve your general level of health. On pages 137–40 you will find a list of Chinese medical and herbal suppliers, where you will be able to obtain materials and herbs required for this home therapy section.

MOXIBUSTION

Moxibustion is the burning of a Chinese herb, Folium Artemisiae Argyii *(Ai Ye)* or mugwort, to treat an area of the body or an acupuncture point. Acupuncture needles basically move the qi but cannot add more qi to the body. Moxibustion, however, both warms the body and adds yang qi to the body. In order for allergies to develop, the defensive qi must be relatively weak as it is defensive qi vacuity that allows wind evils to penetrate the body and disturb the function of the lungs. Self-treatment with moxibustion can be used to supplement the defensive qi of the body and can help prevent invasion by wind evils.

There are several methods of moxibustion. However, the safest, easiest and most effective method for use at home is to use what are called *Ibiki* moxas. These are small, ready-made cones of moxa on self-adhesive platforms manufactured in

Japan. They contain the correct amount of mugwort and the platforms prevent any potential for burning. The adhesive backing prevents the moxa from falling off in the middle of the procedure.

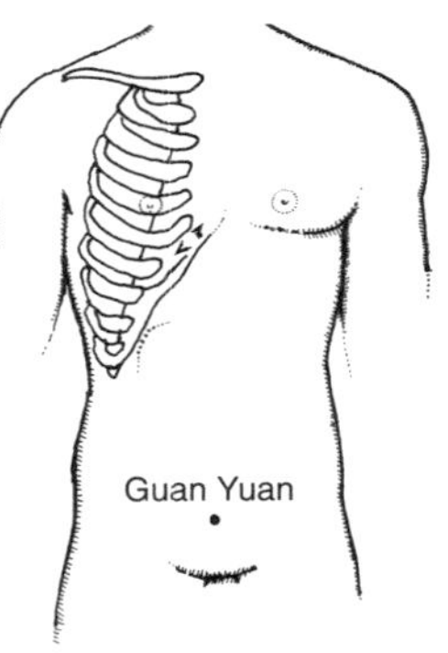

One of the best ways to supplement the yang qi of the body is to moxa two of the most powerful points in the body: *Guan Yuan* (Conception vessel 4) and *Zu San Li* (Stomach 36). *Guan Yuan* is a point on a channel that runs up the centre line of the front of the body, known as the conception vessel. It is located four finger-widths below the navel. This point connects directly to the kidneys, which are the root of all yang in the body. Using moxa on this point invigorates kidney yang, which then supports and fortifies the spleen qi.

Begin by locating this point while lying down on your back in a comfortable position. Stick an Ibiki moxa on the point and light it with a match or lit incense stick. As the moxa cone burns down, if you feel any burning heat lift the cone off the skin. The aim is to turn the skin flushed red and warm under the moxa cone, but not to raise a blister. Only burn one cone the first day. The second day, burn two cones. Add another cone every day (as long as you haven't burned yourself) until you get up to five. Then do this every day for a month before the season you normally experience allergies in. If your allergies are perennial, you may do this at any time of the year, although Chinese medical theory suggests the time between summer and autumn (late summer) is the best time for this therapy. Obviously where you live governs what time of year this season actually falls in, but according to the Chinese medical calendar it begins in the first week of August.

After using moxa on *Guan Yuan,* the next point to do is *Zu San Li.* This is one of the most powerful acupoints on the body. Moxaing this point strongly supplements the spleen and stomach qi. This point is located three finger-widths below the bottom edge of the kneecap on the outside of the lower legs between the tibia and fibula. Place an Ibiki moxa on one *Zu San Li* and burn it in the same way as on *Guan Yuan.*

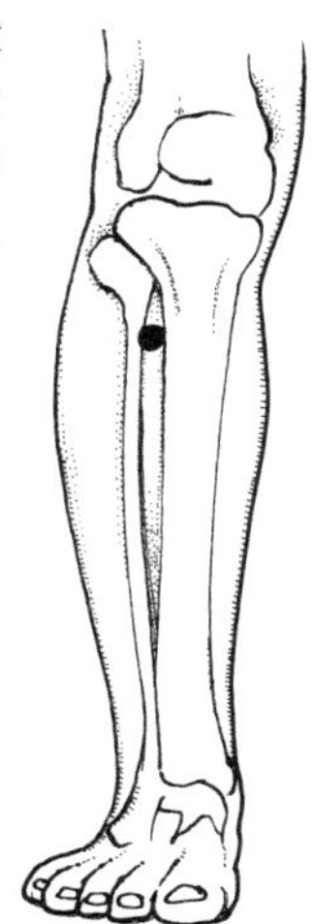

You want a strong heat, but it should not be burning or blistering hot. The first day, only burn one cone. The second day, if all went well, burn two cones. Each day after that, burn three Ibiki cones on *Zu San Li* on each leg.

Always be sure to perform this technique in this order – *Guan Yuan* first and *Zu San Li* second. By combining these two points, you will be supplementing the kidneys and the spleen, the two viscera involved in the production of the defensive qi. If you think you have burned yourself, apply *Ching Hong Wan* burn ointment or, if this is not available, lavender aromatherapy oil is very effective. If you raise a blister, cover this with a sterile dressing and keep clean to avoid infection. Actually, in China, it was once thought that raising a blister meant an even better result would be achieved. If you do raise a blister, let it heal before moxaing again.

This method is for treating the underlying root of most allergies: a spleen-kidney vacuity. It is not for first-aid treatment of allergic rhinitis or asthma during an attack. If the above directions are not sufficiently clear for you to feel confident doing this, go to a professional acupuncturist who can teach you how to locate these points and perform this technique at home.

CUPPING

Cupping is an ancient method of healing dating back to Neolithic times when animal horns were used instead of glass and porcelain cups. Basically, this technique consists of creating a vacuum on the skin which then pulls qi and blood to this area of the body.

In order to do this at home, find an empty glass jar the size of a baby food jar. Hold a small piece of cotton in a pair of pliers, tweezers or forceps. Dip the cotton in a little rubbing alcohol or spirit. Do not get the cotton so wet that it is completely sodden and drips. Lie on your back with your navel exposed. Bring the mouth of the jar down close next to the skin surrounding your navel. Light the alcohol-impregnated cotton ball and quickly place it inside the jar. It will burn out the oxygen and create a vacuum. Pull the cotton ball out of the jar quickly and place the mouth of the jar over the navel. Don't leave the burning cotton in the jar for too long or the jar will be too hot. If you have co-ordinated this correctly, the jar will be stuck to your abdomen with a firm seal. Your navel and the surrounding skin will have been sucked up into the mouth of the jar and the skin should be turning red.

Leave the jar on for three to five minutes and then remove by pressing down on one side of the jar. As soon as air creeps under the edge, the seal will be broken. Do this again three times in succession for a total of 15 minutes. Repeat this every day for 10 days.

This method is a very effective home remedy for treating all kinds of allergies, including allergic rhinitis, asthma and hives. It can be done either before as a preventative measure or during the allergy season in order to eliminate allergic reactions. Again, if these written directions do not seem clear enough for you to feel confident doing this technique, see a professional acupuncturist who can quickly and easily teach you how to do it. It may turn your navel red or even lightly black and blue for a few days, but it really is an effective way for treating allergic conditions. The acupuncture point located in the centre of the navel is connected to both the spleen and the kidneys and supplements both of these at the same time. Cups made in China specifically for this therapy can also be purchased from a Chinese medical supplier.

CHINESE SELF-MASSAGE

Massage, including self-massage, is a highly developed part of traditional Chinese medicine. In most traditional Chinese hospitals, there are massage wards where patients can receive treatment for almost every disease. The following Chinese self-massage regime can be used to treat acute cases of allergic rhinitis with a runny nose, nasal congestion and sore, red, itchy eyes.

1. Opening heaven's gate

Push upwards with the index and middle fingers of both hands along the midline of the forehead from the midpoint between the eyebrows to the anterior hairline. Begin at the level of the eyebrows and alternately push upwards to the hairline again and again, 50–100 times, pushing in one direction only, from the eyebrows upward to the hairline.

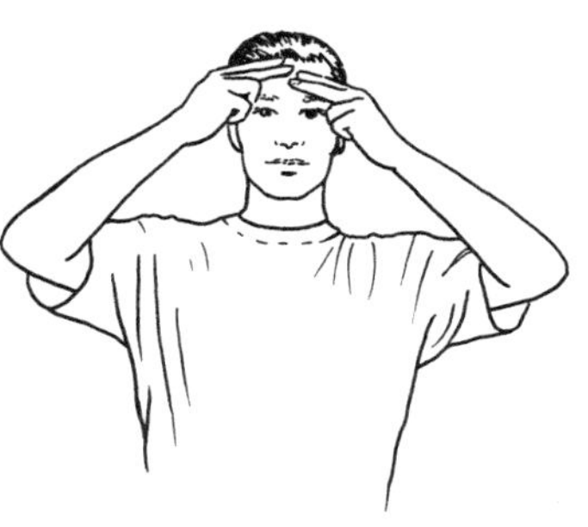

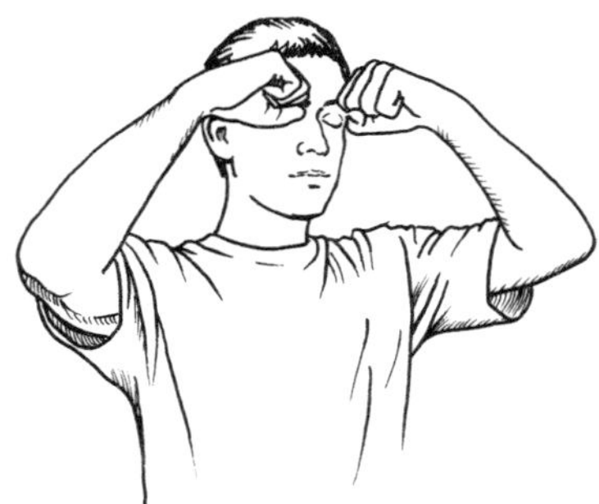

2. Pushing apart the forehead
Bend the two index fingers and push with the lateral sides of their middle segments from the midline of the forehead to the anterior hairline on both sides of the forehead and the ends of the eyebrows. Do this approximately 100 times.

3. Kneading *Tai Yang*
Press with the tip of the thumbs or middle fingers on the points *Tai Yang* located in the centre of each temple. Knead them approximately 100 times until there is a sensation of mild soreness and distension.

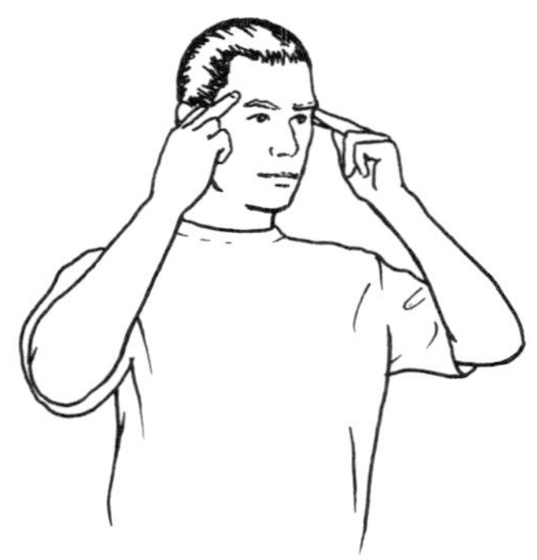

4. Wiping the temples
Press the temples with the pads of the thumbs and wipe backwards repeatedly with force approximately 100 times until there is a sensation of mild soreness and distension.

5. Pressing and kneading *Feng Chi* (Gall Bladder 20)

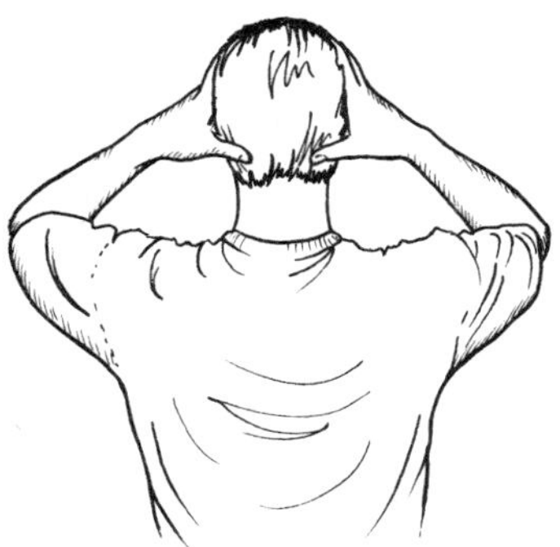

With the tips of both thumbs, press and knead the paired points *Feng Chi,* located in the depression between the upper portion of the sternocleido-mastoid muscles and the trapezius, approximately 2.5 cm/ 1 in into the hairline; do this100 times. The force should be strong enough to make the forehead sweat.

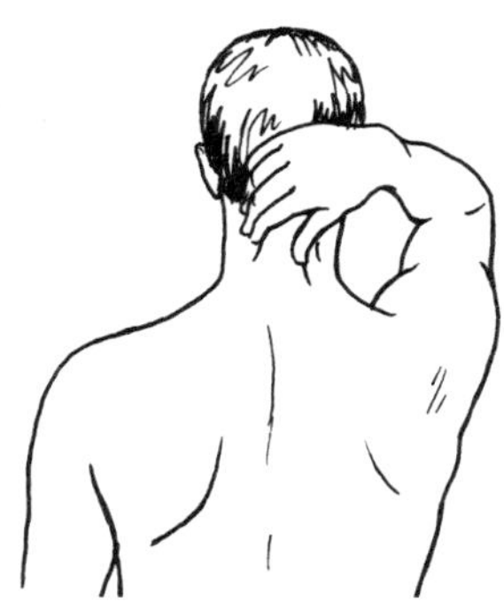

6. Grasping the muscles on both sides of the nape of the neck

Put the thumb of one hand on one side of the nape of the neck and the index and middle fingers on the other, grasping the muscles of both sides from the posterior hairline to the base of the neck 10–20 times.

7. Grasping and pounding *Jian Jing* (Gall Bladder 21)

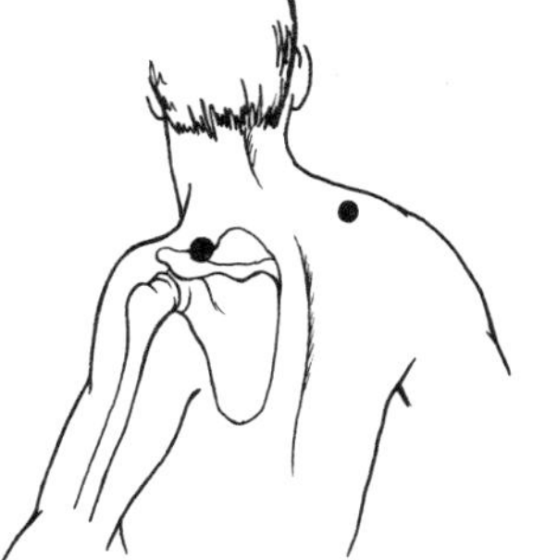

With the thumb, index and middle fingers of the left hand, grasp the right *Jian Jing,* located at the midpoint of the top of the shoulder muscle, 3–5 times. Then switch hands and grasp the left *Jian Jing* with the right hand. Next, pound the point with a loosely closed fist 30–50 times on each side.

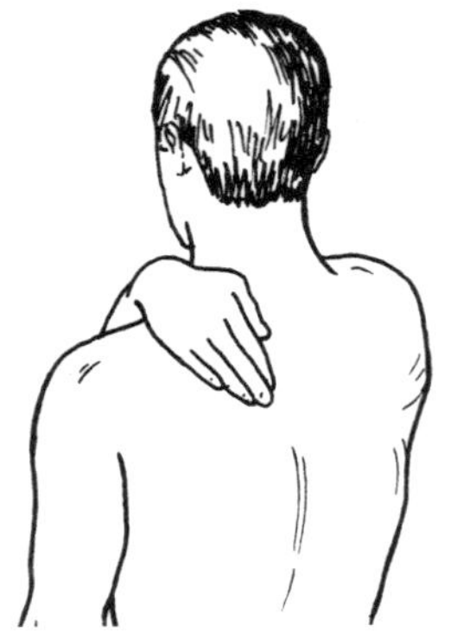

8. Patting the back

With a cupped palm, pat the opposite side of the upper back 30–50 times on each side.

9. Nipping and kneading *He Gu* (Large intestine 4)

With the nail of the opposite thumb, nip and knead the point *He Gu*, located at the midpoint of the mound of muscle between the thumb and index finger on the back of the hand, approximately 100 times each side.

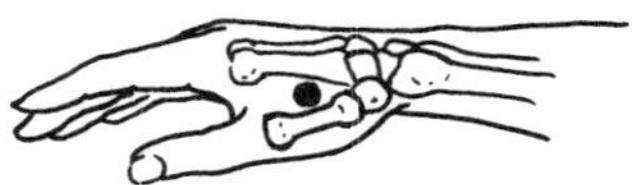

10. Kneading *Ying Xiang* (Large intestine 20)

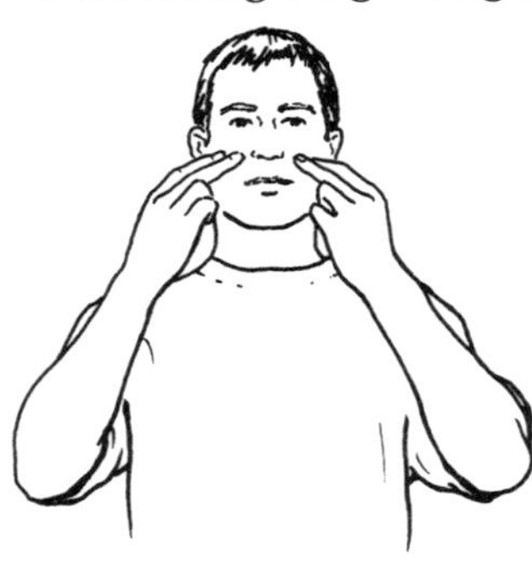

Knead the points on either side of the wings of the nose with the tips of the middle fingers approximately 100 times. This treatment is for use during an acute allergic attack. Even just the last two manoeuvres can be helpful in relieving the symptoms of an acute allergic episode.

In order to supplement the spleen and kidneys, the underlying root of most respiratory allergies, this next regime can be done daily between allergic attacks.

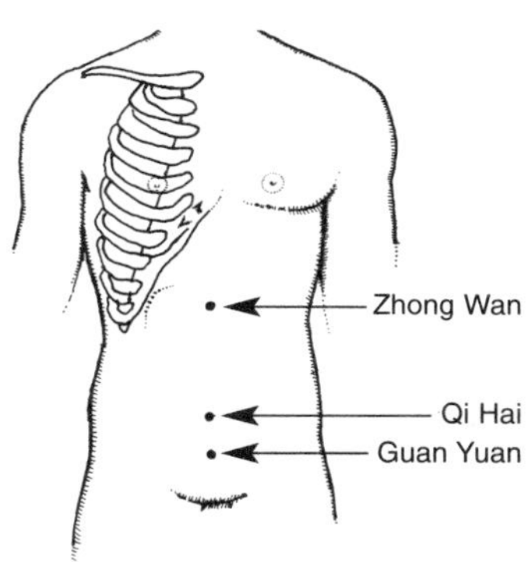

1. Pressing and kneading *Zhong Wan* (Conception vessel 12), *Qi Hai* (Conception vessel 6) and *Guan Yuan* (Conception vessel 4)

With one palm, press and knead the midpoint of the upper abdomen, the point 4 cm/1½ in below the navel and the midpoint of the lower abdomen, approximately 100 times each.

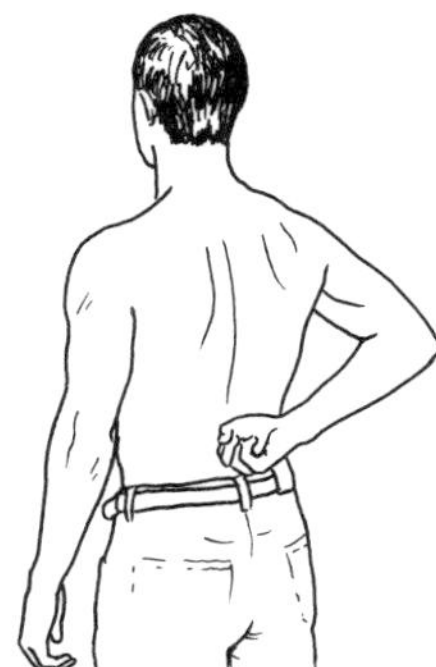

2. Pounding the lumbar region

With loosely clenched fists, pound the entire lower back region, the mansion of the kidneys, 30–50 times.

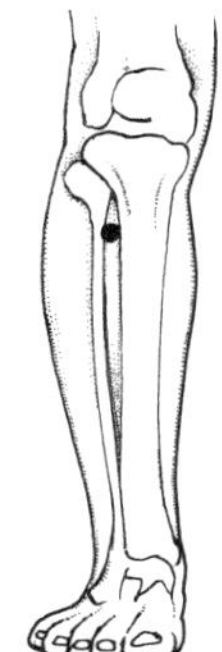

3. Pressing and kneading *Zu San Li* (Stomach 36)

With the tips of both thumbs, press and knead *Zu San Li*, located 8 cm/3 in below the lower outside corner of the kneecap, approximately 100 times each.

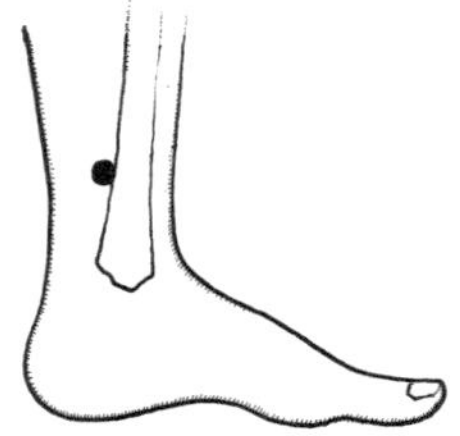

4. Pressing and kneading *San Yin Jiao* (Spleen 6)
With the tips of both thumbs, press and knead the points located 8 cm/3 in above the tip of the inner ankles just behind the tibia, 50–100 times each.

The key to getting a positive effect from Chinese self-massage in terms of building up one's bodily constitution is persevering with daily practice. Even just rubbing the abdomen after meals can improve the spleen and stomach function. For more Chinese self-massage regimes, the reader should see *Fan Ya-li's Chinese Self-massage Therapy: The Easy Way to Health* (see page 153).

SEVEN STAR HAMMERING

A seven star hammer is a small hammer or mallet with seven small needles embedded in its head. This is one way to stimulate acupuncture points without inserting a needle into the body. It is also an excellent method to move congested qi. Seven star hammers can be useful for those who are frightened of needles and for children, as well as for home therapy treatment. When the points to be stimulated are located on the front of the body you may do the treatment yourself. You will, however, need to get someone to assist if the points are located on the back of the body.

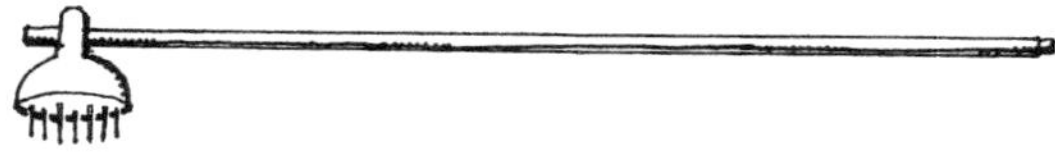

This is a very easy technique which does not require any special training or expertise.

During an acute attack of allergic rhinitis or asthma, begin by tapping the nape of the neck, tapping most tbetween the second and fourth cervical vertebrae. Also tap the region of *Feng Chi* (Gall Bladder 20). This point is located behind the ears, just below the base of the skull in the depression between the strap muscles of the spine and the attachment of the sternocleidomastoid muscles at the mastoid process.

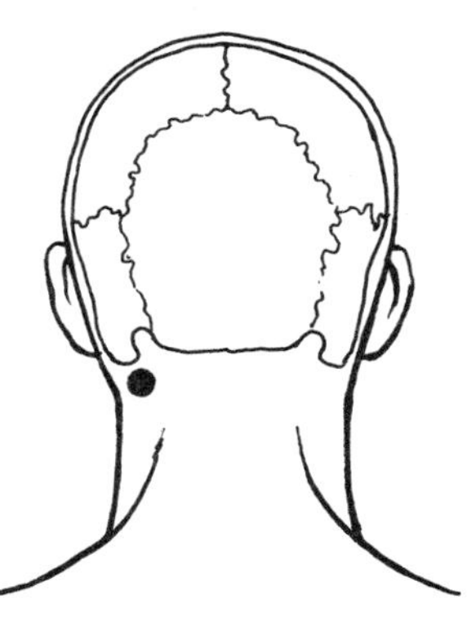

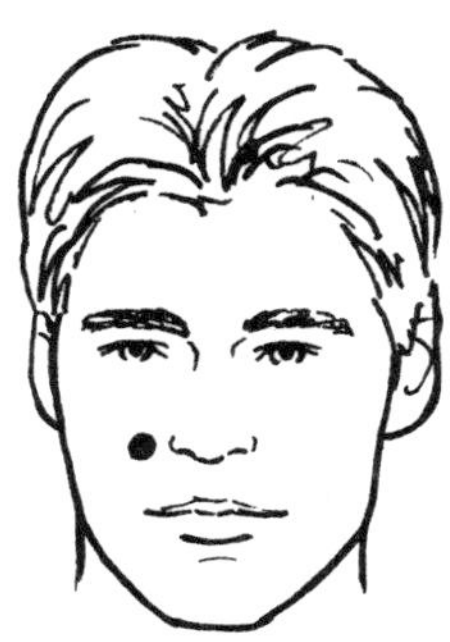

Then tap *Ying Xiang* (Large intestine 20) on both sides of the wings of the nose.

Follow this by tapping *He Gu* (Large intestine 4). This point is located in the centre of the mound between the thumb and index finger on the back of the hand.

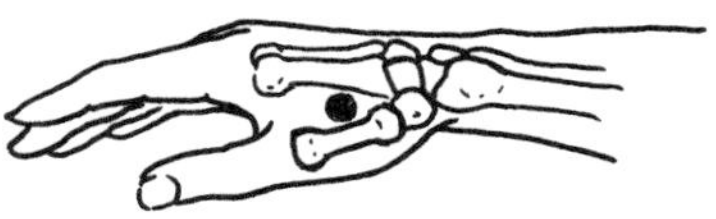

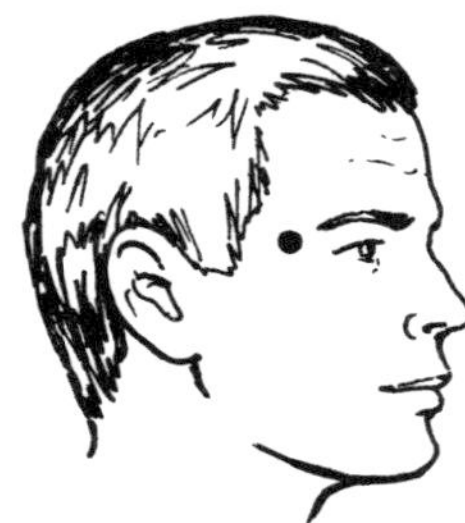

If there are red, itchy, painful eyes or headache, tap *Tai Yang*. This point is located right in the centre of the temple.

If there is asthma, add the entire upper back region between the spine and inside edges of the shoulder blades, the front and back intercostal spaces, both sides of the trachea or windpipe, the lower edge of the zyphoid process just below the centre of the ribs and *Tai Yuan* (Lungs 9). This point is located at the wrist crease on the outside edge of the radial artery where the pulse is felt. Use moderate to heavy tapping.

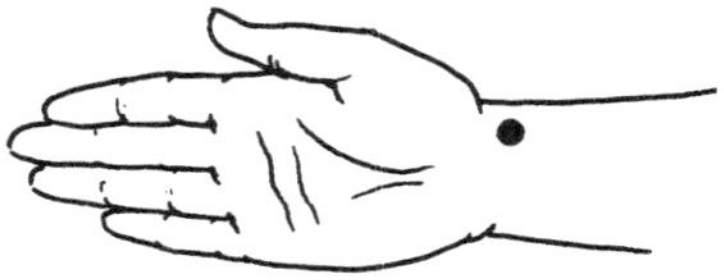

If there is any bleeding, wipe the area with a cotton swab moistened in alcohol. Then take a dry cotton ball and press the area.

To strengthen the system between allergic attacks, one can tap the following areas more lightly once per day or once every other day:

1. Both sides of the entire spinal column from the sacrum to the base of the skull.

2. *Zhong Wan* (Conception vessel 12): The centre of the upper abdomen.

3. *Qi Hai* (Conception vessel 6): 4 cm/1½ in below the navel on the midline of the lower abdomen.

4. *Guan Yuan* (Conception vessel 4): The centre of the lower abdomen.

5. *Zu San Li* (Stomach 36): 8 cm/3 in below the lower, outer corner of the kneecap.

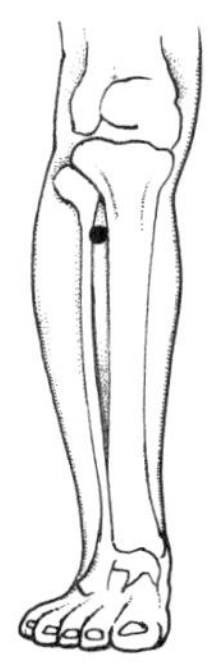

Between treatments, soak the seven star hammer in alcohol or hydrogen peroxide. In order to prevent infection, always use your own personal hammer – do not share with anyone else.

CHINESE HERBAL REMEDIES FOR HOME THERAPY

In this next section I will give you some recipes which you can make at home in the form of porridges and teas. As with all Chinese herbs, I strongly recommend that you seek professional guidance with regard to their usage. Should you choose to try one of these recipes and notice any unwanted side-effects, stop taking it immediately and seek professional advice.

Chinese medicinal porridges

Chinese medicinal porridges are a specialised part of Chinese dietary therapy. Porridges are very easily digestible since they already take the form of a 100°F soup and they are a particularly good way of eating nutritious grains which could otherwise be difficult to digest. When Chinese medicinals are cooked together with grains in the form of a porridge, this makes a high-powered and easily assimilated nutritious 'health food' of the first order. Eating soups and porridges is predigestion and this helps a vacuous, weak spleen. Medicinal porridges can be used to treat acute attacks of allergic rhinitis and asthma, and to build up the system and treat the root in between attacks. In English, such Chinese medicinal porridges are often referred to as congees.

Jie Cai Zhou **(Mustard Greens Congee)**

60 g/2¼ oz	Fresh mustard greens, i.e. Herba Sinapis Junceae *(Jie Cai)*
100 g/4 oz	Polished rice, i.e. Semen Oryzae Sativae *(Jing Mi)*

First wash and cut the mustard greens. Then cook these and the rice in water to make into a dilute rice soup. Eat warm twice a day. This formula is for the treatment of cold phlegm cough and asthma, the phlegm being clear and watery, as it often is in most cases of simple allergic rhinitis. It diffuses the lungs, clears away phlegm and boosts the stomach.

Su Ye Xing Ren Zhou **(Perilla Leaf and Apricot Seed Congee)**

9 g	Folium Perillae Frutescentis *(Zi Su Ye)*
9 g	Semen Pruni Armeniacae *(Xing Ren)*
6 g	Pericarpium Citri Reticulatae *(Chen Pi)*
50 g/2 oz	Polished rice, i.e. Semen Oryzae Sativae *(Jing Mi)*

Boil the first three ingredients in water, strain off the dregs and add the remaining liquid to the rice. Cook the rice into porridge with this liquid and eat. This formula is for wind cold rhinitis, bronchitis and asthma. It resolves the exterior, transforms phlegm, moves and corrects the flow of qi and stops coughing and sneezing. If you don't have all four ingredients, you can still make a medicinal congee with only the last three or even just the Semen Pruni and rice.

Hu Tao Zhou **(Walnut Congee)**

50 g/2 oz Walnuts, i.e. Semen Juglandis Regiae *(Hu Tao Ren)*
50 g/2 oz Polished rice, i.e. Semen Oryzae Sativae *(Jing Mi)*

Pound the walnuts into a mash and add water to the rice and cook into porridge. After the porridge is cooked, add the walnut mash and mix thoroughly. Skim off any oil on the top of the porridge and eat the congee warm once each morning and evening. This formula supplements the kidneys, boosts the lungs and stabilises panting, i.e. asthma and coughing. It can be used to treat the root of lung, spleen, kidney allergic rhinitis and asthma. It is not suitable for first-aid use during an acute attack.

Chong Cao Zhou **(Cordyceps Congee)**

6 g Cordyceps Sinensis *(Dong Chong Xia Cao)*
50 g/2 oz Polished rice, i.e. Semen Oryzae Sativae *(Jing Mi)*

First cook the rice into porridge. Powder the Cordyceps and add to the cooked congee. Mix thoroughly and cook for a little longer. Eat warm twice a day. Five to seven days is one course of treatment. This formula boosts the lungs and supplements the kidneys, enriches yin and stops panting, i.e. asthma. It benefits the lungs, spleen and kidneys, and helps both allergic rhinitis and asthma.

For further Chinese medicinal porridge formulae for respiratory problems and asthma, see *The Book of Jook: Chinese Medicinal Porridges* (see page 154).

Chinese medicinal teas

When patients go to a professional practitioner of Chinese medicine, they will usually come away with a herbal formula with a dozen or more ingredients. They will probably have to boil these ingredients into a very strong decoction for

45–60 minutes or more. Medicinal teas, however, do not require as much preparation and are not as strong and powerful medicinally as a decoction. They are really considered to be more folk remedies than Chinese herbal medicine. If you do choose to try them unsupervised, take care and stop immediately should you experience any adverse effects. Since they are for the relief of the symptoms of an acute attack of allergic rhinitis you will not be taking them for a long period of time anyway.

Cang Er Zi Cha **(Xanthium Tea)**

12 g Fructus Xanthii Sibirici *(Cang Er Zi)*
6 g Flos Magnoliae Liliflorae *(Xin Yi Hua)*
6 g Radix Angelicae Dahuricae *(Bai Zhi)*
6 g Herba Menthae Haplocalycis *(Bo He)*
2 g Tea leaves, i.e. Folium Camelliae Theae *(Cha Ye)*

Grind these five ingredients into powder and steep in boiling water for 10 minutes. This amount of powder should provide enough for one day. Drink the tea warm at any time throughout the day. This formula resolves the exterior, dispels wind, opens the portals of the nose and eliminates dampness.

Xin Yi Cha **(Magnolia Flower Tea)**

2 g Flos Magnoliae Liliflorae *(Xin Yi Hua)*
6 g Folium Perillae Frutescentis *(Zi Su Ye)*

Grind the two ingredients into a coarse powder, wrap in muslin (cheesecloth) or put in a tea infuser and soak in boiling water. Drink this as a tea during the course of the day. This formula dispels wind, scatters cold and frees the portals of the nose.

Bai Zhi Jing Jie Cha (Angelica and Schizonepeta Tea)

30 g/1 oz	Radix Angelicae Dahuricae *(Bai Zhi)*
3 g	Herba Seu Flos Schizonepetae Tenuifoliae *(Jing Jie Sui)*
3 g	Tea leaves, i.e. Folium Camelliae Theae *(Cha Ye)*

Grind the first two ingredients into a fine powder. Steep the tea leaves in boiling water. Using this beverage, wash down 6g of the powder twice a day. This formula dispels wind and scatters cold, resolves the exterior and stops pain. It treats wind cold external invasions with nasal congestion, clear nasal mucus and headache, where headache is a major symptom.

Ju Hua Long Jing Cha (Chrysanthemum and Dragon Well Tea)

10 g	Flos Chrysanthemi Morifolii *(Ju Hua)*
3 g	Dragon Well Tea, i.e. Folium Camelliae Theae *(Long Jing Cha)*

Steep these two ingredients in boiling water for 5–10 minutes. This quantity is enough for one day, drunk as a tea at any time. This formula treats red, itchy eyes caused by a combination of wind and heat.

The next two Chinese folk teas are for treating the underlying root of respiratory allergies and asthma. The first is designed to help eliminate phlegm dampness. The second is to supplement the spleen and kidneys and thus prevent asthma due to spleen-kidney vacuity weakness. These teas can be drunk over a longer time period as they are not aimed at relieving acute symptoms.

Ju Cha (Tangerine Tea)

2 g Tea leaves, i.e. Folium Camelliae Theae *(Cha Ye)*
2 g Dry tangerine peel, i.e. Pericarpium Citri Reticulatae *(Ju Pi)*

Place these two ingredients in a cup, pour in boiling water and steep for 10 minutes. This tea stops coughing, transforms phlegm, rectifies the qi and harmonises the stomach. Frequent drinking of this tea can help reduce or eliminate phlegm dampness.

Ren Shen Hu Tao Cha (Ginseng and Walnut Tea)

4 g Radix Panacis Ginseng *(Ren Shen)*
4 halves of walnut, i.e. Semen Juglandis Regiae *(Hu Tao Ren)*

Pound the ginseng and walnuts into pieces, place them in a pot and boil with water over a slow fire. This should make 400 ml/14 fl oz of concentrated liquid. Drink this amount per day, taken at any time. The ginseng and walnut can also be chewed and eaten. This tea fortifies the spleen, supplements the kidneys, absorbs the qi[2] and reduces panting. This formula is suitable for treating the root of chronic asthma due to spleen–kidney vacuity. It is used between acute attacks in order to 'bank the root', i.e. strengthen the body.

For more information on Chinese medicinal teas, see *Chinese Medicinal Teas: Simple, Proven Folk Formulas for Common Diseases and Promoting Health* (see page 156).

[2] In Chinese medicine, the kidneys grasp or absorb the qi sent down by the lungs on inhalation. Asthma due to kidney vacuity is due, at least in part, to the kidneys being too weak to grasp or absorb this qi, which then counterflows back upwards as panting or coughing.

CREATING A PERSONAL REGIME

It is not necessary to use all these home treatments if you are suffering from hay fever. Choose several of them that appeal to you and are manageable. The more severe your condition, the more support you are likely to need. It is best to make sure you first use the three 'free' therapies and then add these home remedies depending on what you can best manage.

CHINESE MEDICAL RESEARCH ON RESPIRATORY ALLERGIES

Considerable research has been done in the People's Republic of China into the effects of acupuncture and Chinese herbal medicine on allergic rhinitis and asthma. Usually, this research is in the form of a clinical audit. That means that a group of patients with the same diseases, patterns or major complaints are given the same treatment for a certain period of time. After this time, the patients are assessed to see how many are cured, how many show a marked improvement and how many had no result. This kind of 'outcome-based research' has, until only very recently, not been considered credible in the West where, for the last 30 years or so, the double-blind, placebo-controlled comparison study has been considered the 'gold standard'. However, such double-blind, placebo-controlled comparison studies are impossible to design in Chinese medicine and do not, in any case, measure the effectiveness of the treatment in a real-life situation.

Clinical audits, on the other hand, do measure actual clinical satisfaction of real-life patients. Such clinical audits may not exclude the patient's trust and belief in the therapist or the therapy itself as an important component in the result. Real life is not as neat and discrete as a controlled laboratory experiment. But if the majority of patients are satisfied with the results of a particular treatment and there are no adverse side-effects to it, then as far as I am concerned it is good enough for me and, in my experience, it is good enough for the vast majority of my patients.

Below are abbreviated translations of several recent research articles published in Chinese medical journals demonstrating how Chinese medicine treats allergic rhinitis and asthma. I think that most people reading these statistics might think that Chinese medicine is worth a try. Still better results can be expected when treatments are even more finely tuned to the individual patient as is the case in private practice here in the West.

Treatment Research 1

From 'The Treatment of 42 Cases of Allergic Rhinitis with *Si Wu Tang Jia Wei* (Four Materials Decoction with Added Flavours)' by Li Guang-zhen, Ji Lin Zhong Yi Yao (Jilin Chinese Medicine and Medicinals), No. 3, 1993

Since 1985, the author has treated 42 cases of allergic rhinitis with *Si Wu Tang Jia Wei.* Of these 42 cases, 29 were men and 13 were women. They ranged in age from 19 to 62 years. The shortest duration of disease was four months and the longest was 10 years. Runny nose, itchy nose and sneezing were the main symptoms. Examination revealed that the nasal mucosa were either an ashen white or purplish, sooty colour, the soft tissue inside the nose was swollen with fluid and it was producing a flowing secretion. Examination of the nasal secretions were positive for eosinophils (a type of white blood cell involved in allergy and inflammation).

Treatment method

The medicinals consisted of:

24 g/1 oz	Uncooked Radix Rehmanniae *(Sheng Di)*
15 g/½ oz	Radix Angelicae Sinensis *(Dang Gui)*
15 g/½ oz	Radix Rubrus Paeoniae Lactiflorae *(Chi Shao)*
6 g	Radix Ligustici Wallichii *(Chuan Xiong)*
9 g	Fructus Xanthii *(Cang Er Zi)*
9 g	Flos Magnoliae Liliflorae *(Xin Yi)*

30 g/1 oz Herba Pycnostelmae *(Xu Chang Jing)*

If there was headache, Radix Angelicae Dahuricae *(Bai Zhi)* and Flos Chrysanthemi Morifolii *(Ju Hua)* were added.

If there was a common cold, these medicinals were combined with *Yu Ping Feng San* (Jade Windscreen Powder).

One *ji*[3] was decocted each day with one course of treatment lasting 15 days. Two to four courses of treatment were given with a follow-up survey conducted one year after treatment.

Treatment outcomes

Out of 42 patients, 23 were completely cured. This meant that their symptoms disappeared, their nasal mucosa and secretions returned to normal and their nasal secretions tested negative for eosinophils. A further 13 cases showed a fair improvement. This meant that their symptoms were obviously reduced or partially disappeared. The number or duration of attacks was also reduced and the nasal secretions of the majority tested negative for eosinophils. Six patients got no result from this treatment. This meant that there was no apparent change in their condition from before the treatment was begun. Therefore, overall, the effectiveness rate was 85.7 per cent.

Discussion

According to the author, the main Chinese medicine disease mechanism of this disease is yin and blood insufficiency. In that case, constructive and defensive are empty and sparse and the exterior defensive fails to secure. Her basic defences

---

[3] *Ji* literally means a prescription. However, when used as it is in these research reports, a ji means a single packet of medicinals, the doses of whose ingredients have been given above. Usually, one ji is a one-day dose. However, because this is typically given in two or more divided doses, to translate this word as dose could be ambiguous.

and energies are depleted and insufficient so she is prone to illness and infection. This then allows for external invasion of wind cold and this results in the portals of the lungs losing their disinhibition (i.e. the nose is runny and blocked with mucus). *Si Wu Tang* enriches yin and nourishes blood, moves the qi and harmonises the constructive, thus supporting the righteous. As the saying goes, 'When the blood is harmonious (or harmonised), wind is automatically extinguished.' Xanthium, Flos Magnoliae and Pynostelma diffuse the lungs, open the portals and therefore dispel evils. When evils are dispelled, the righteous is at ease. With the righteous returned and evils removed, the disease obtains a cure.

Treatment Research 2

From 'The Treatment of 100 Cases of Allergic Rhinitis with *Bu Zhong Yi Qi Tang Jia Wei* (Supplement the Centre and Boost the Qi Decoction with Added Flavours)' by Feng Bi-qun and Lu Ji-sen, Xin Zhong Yi (*New Chinese Medicine*), No. 6, 1995

Since 1988, the authors have treated 100 patients suffering from allergic rhinitis with *Bu Zhong Yi Qi Tang Jia Wei* with good success. Of those 100 patients, 62 were males and 38 were females. The youngest was 13 and the oldest was 58 years old with most cases falling between 16 and 40. The disease course had lasted for less than one year in 17 cases, for one to 10 years in 77 cases and for more than 10 years in six cases. The clinical manifestations were recurrent sneezing, runny nose, nasal congestion and nasal itching. Examination of the nasal mucosa revealed that they were oedematous, coloured a sombre white or an ashen grey and that there was usually a great amount of clear, watery mucus.

Treatment method

The formula comprised:

Radix Astragali Membranacei *(Huang Qi)*
Radix Codonopsitis Pilosulae *(Dang Shen)*
Mix-fried Radix Glycyrrhizae *(Zhi Gan Cao)*
Rhizoma Atractylodis Macrocephalae *(Bai Zhu)*
Pericarpium Citri Reticulatae *(Chen Pi)*
Radix Angelicae Sinensis *(Dang Gui)*
Rhizoma Cimicifugae *(Sheng Ma)*
Radix Bupleuri *(Chai Hu)*
Fructus Xanthii Sibirici *(Cang Er Zi)*
Flos Magnoliae Liliflorae *(Xin Yi Hua)*

The doses of these ingredients depended upon what was appropriate for the individual, and the formula was modified following the patterns.

If there was an exterior pattern, Radix Ledebouriellae Divaricatae *(Fang Feng)*, fresh Bulbus Allii Fistulosi *(Cong Bai)* and Semen Praeparatus Sojae *(Dan Dou Chi)* were added.

If yang vacuity was marked, Radix Lateralis Praeparatus Aconiti Carmichaeli *(Fu Zi)*, Herba Epimedii *(Yin Yang Huo)* and Fructus Rosae Laevigatae *(Jin Ying Zi)* were added.

If there was simultaneous yin vacuity, Herba Dendrobii *(Shi Hu)*, Rhizoma Polygoni Odorati *(Yu Zhu)* and Fructus Ligustri Lucidi *(Nu Zhen Zi)* were added.

Definition of treatment outcomes

Complete cure was defined as the disappearance of sneezing, runny nose, nasal congestion, nasal itching and other such symptoms. There was no oedema of the nasal passageways and no inflammatory secretion. After one year there was no relapse.

Some effect was defined as marked decrease in the symptoms, no obvious nasal mucosal oedema or inflammatory secretion, but recurrence once in a while in the next year.

No effect meant that there was no obvious change from before to after treatment.

Treatment outcomes

Based on the above criteria, there were 62 cures with another 30 patients showing some effect. Eight cases experienced no results from this protocol. Thus, overall, the effectiveness rate was 92 per cent.

Discussion

According to the authors, allergic rhinitis is a commonly seen disease with a long duration and is difficult to cure. In Chinese medicine, it is categorised as runny mucus disorder. Due to lung qi vacuity, wind cold pathogens lodge in the nasal cavity. The lung qi loses its free flow and fluids and humours collect and gather. The nasal cavity becomes congested and blocked and therefore there is sneezing and a runny nose. However, the repletion and fullness of the lung qi is dependent on the transportation of the spleen qi. Therefore, *Bu Zhong Yi Qi Tang* is used to fortify the spleen and boost the qi, move up the clear and transform dampness. Boosting the spleen energies helps, in turn, to boost the lung energies. Xanthium and Flos Magnoliae are added to assist in scattering wind and cold, opening and disinhibiting the portal of the lungs, i.e. unblocking the nose and sinuses. This then strengthens and increases the treatment effect.

Treatment Research 3

From 'The Treatment of 65 Cases of Allergic Rhinitis with *Jia Jian Xiao Chai Hu Tang* (Modified Minor Bupleurum Decoction)' by Kuang Nai-jia, Bi Guo-mei and Huang Ya-shan, He Nan Zhong Yi *(Henan Chinese Medicine)*, No. 5, 1995

From January 1991 to July 1993, the authors treated 65 cases of allergic rhinitis with modified *Xiao Chai Hu Tang* with very good results. They began with a group of 130 patients and divided them in half into treatment and comparison groups. Of the 65 patients in the treatment group, 35 were men and 30 were women. They ranged in age from 18 to 65 years old and their disease course had lasted from one to nine years. Ten patients had a mild degree of disease, 25 a moderate degree and 30 patients had a severe degree of disease. In the comparison group, there were 36 men and 29 women. They ranged in age from 17 to 66 years old and they had been ill for between one and 10 years. Nine patients in that group had a mild degree of disease, 26 a moderate degree and 30 a severe degree of disease. Thus these two groups were very similar statistically.

Treatment method

Xiao Chai Hu Tang consisted of:

12 g/½ oz	Radix Bupleuri *(Chai Hu)*
9 g	Radix Scutellariae Baicalensis *(Huang Qin)*
6 g	Radix Panacis Ginseng *(Ren Shen)*
6 g	Mix-fried Radix Glycyrrhizae *(Zhi Gan Cao)*
3 slices	Uncooked Rhizoma Zingiberis *(Sheng Jiang)*
4 pieces	Fructus Zizyphi Jujubae *(Da Zao)*

One *ji* was decocted in water each day and given warm in two divided doses. This was continued for four weeks.

If there was nasal itching and especially heavy sneezing, Flos Magnoliae Liliflorae *(Xin Yi Hua)* and Flos Chrysanthemi Morifolii *(Ju Hua)* were added.

If there was relatively profuse runny nose with clear mucus, Rhizoma Atractylodis *(Cang Zhu)* and Rhizoma Cimicifugae *(Sheng Ma)* were added.

If the soft tissue inside the nose was markedly swollen and distended, Radix Angelicae Dahuricae *(Bai Zhi)* and Herba Menthae Haplocalycis *(Bo He)* were added.

If the nasal cavity was red and blood-filled and particularly inflamed, Rhizoma Coptidis Chinensis *(Huang Lian)* and Radix Ligustici Wallichii *(Chuan Xiong)* were added.

If there were polyps in the nasal conchae, Semen Pruni Persicae *(Tao Ren)* and Radix Puerariae *(Ge Gen)* were added.

If there was accompanying accessory nasal sinusitis, Radix Salviae Miltiorrhizae *(Dan Shen)* and Rhizoma Coptidis Chinensis *(Huang Lian)* were added.

If there was accompanying headache, Rhizoma Ligustici Wallichii *(Chuan Xiong)* and Radix Et Rhizoma Ligustici Chinensis *(Gao Ben)* were added.

If there were accompanying itchy, watery eyes and inflammation of the conjunctiva around the eyes, Radix Astragali Membranacei *(Huang Qi)*, Flos Chrysanthemi Morifolii *(Ju Hua)* and Radix Ledebouriellae Divaricatae *(Fang Feng)* were added.

If there was accompanying bronchial asthma, Cortex Radicis Mori Albi *(Sang Bai Pi)* and Radix Platycodi Grandiflori *(Jie Geng)* were added.

If there was accompanying tinnitus, ear oppression, or deafness, Radix Angelicae Sinensis *(Dang Gui)*, Rhizoma Alismatis *(Ze Xie)* and Rhizoma Acori Graminei *(Chang Pu)* were added.

The comparison group was given 4 mg of chlorpheniramine three times each day. At the same time, both groups used Benadryl[4] liquid nose drops. No other systemic medicinals were used.

---

[4] Benadryl is an American drug brand name, now discontinued in the UK.

Treatment outcomes

Effectiveness was based on subjective changes in sneezing, runny nose and nasal obstruction as well as on objective changes in the nasal mucosa. Of the treatment group, 34 cases experienced marked effect, 25 some effect and 6 no effect. Thus the total effectiveness of this protocol in the treatment group was 90.8 per cent. Of these patients, 59 were followed up after two years and only seven of these, or 11.9 per cent, had a recurrence. In the comparison group, 29 experienced marked effect, 21 some effect and 15 no effect, for an overall effectiveness rate of 76.9 per cent. Of these patients, 50 were followed up after two years and 16 cases, or 32 per cent, had relapses. Thus there was a marked statistical difference between these two groups in terms of the effectiveness of protocols and also their relapse rates. Therefore, *Xiao Chai Hu Tang* is obviously more effective than chlorpheniramine. Tests also showed that the levels of immunoglobins found in nasal secretions were improved after treatment with *Xiao Chai Hu Tang.*

Discussion

According to the authors, allergic rhinitis is due to spleen–lung qi vacuity and poor defence mechanisms. Thus wind cold takes advantage of vacuity and enters, assailing and harassing the nasal cavity. Hence the main branch symptoms are nasal itching, sneezing, clear mucus, runny nose and nasal obstruction. According to Japanese research reported by Zhang Zhi-jun in *Zhong Yi Za Zhi (Journal of Chinese Medicine)* No. 10, 1993, *Xiao Chai Hu Tang* has relatively strong anti-allergy, anti-inflammatory and immune function strengthening abilities. Therefore it can treat both the branch and the root simultaneously. Within this formula, Bupleurum clears heat and resolves the exterior. Hence, pathogens are released to the outside. Scutellaria clears heat and dries dampness. When combined with Bupleurum, it externally percolates and internally clears, expels cold and removes evils. Ginseng and red dates open the network vessels and quicken the blood, fortify the spleen and supplement the qi, support the righteous and dispel evils and protect against evils being transmitted internally. Uncooked ginger and liquorice regulate cold and heat, harmonise the constructive and defensive, clear heat, resolve toxins and open the portals. According to modern medical theory, Bupleurum, Scutellaria, ginseng, liquorice, uncooked ginger and red dates reduce infection and fever. They are anti-inflammatory and anti-allergic and increase the body's immune function. They also improve microcirculation, increasing the volume of blood flow, while decreasing inflammatory reactions affecting the capillaries. Typically, after administering this formula for two weeks, nasal itching, sneezing, clear runny nose and nasal obstruction were all markedly diminished and the inflammatory reactions of the nasal cavity had obviously disappeared. Since the effectiveness rate is high, the recurrence rate is low, there is no particular toxicity and both root and branch are treated simultaneously, *Xiao Chai Hu Tang* is an effective formula for the treatment of allergic rhinitis.

Treatment Research 4

From 'The Treatment of Allergic Rhinitis Mainly by Moxibustion' by Zhang Gui-rong *et al.*, *Zhong Guo Zhen Jiu (Chinese National Acupuncture and Moxibustion)*, No. 4, 1995

There were 135 patients in this clinical audit. Of these, 75 were men and 60 were women. They ranged in age from seven to 58 years. However, the majority of these patients were under 20 years old. The disease duration was as short as four months to as long as 20 years. Treatment lasted from 10 to 40 days.

Treatment method

The points chosen consisted of: *Yin Tang, Zu San Li* (Stomach 36), *He Gu* (Large intestine 4) and *Fei Shu* (Bladder 13). These were treated by indirect moxibustion carried out on top of slices of uncooked Rhizoma Zingiberis *(Jiang Pian)*. These were cut as thick as a coin and a needle was used to poke holes in these. Each point was moxaed with three cones until the skin was flushed red. The points were treated once a day, with 10 days equalling one course of treatment.

Chinese medicinals consisted of:

Wine (stir-fried) Radix Scutellariae Baicalensis *(Jiu Qin)*
Rhizoma Atractylodis *(Cang Zhu)*
Rhizoma Pinelliae Ternatae *(Ban Xia)*
Flos Magnoliae Liliflorae *(Xin Yi)*
Radix Ligustici Wallichii *(Chuan Xiong)*
Radix Angelicae Dahuricae *(Bai Zhi)*
Gypsum Fibrosum *(Shi Gao)*
Radix Panacis Ginseng *(Ren Shen)*
Radix Puerariae *(Ge Gen)*

One *ji* of these was decocted in water and administered each day with a continuous administration of seven days.

Definition of treatment outcomes

Cure meant that the clinical symptoms completely disappeared and one year later there had been no recurrence. Fair or good effect meant that the greater part of the clinical symptoms had disappeared and, although there was recurrence, the symptoms were reduced. No effect meant that there was no change in the clinical symptoms.

Treatment outcomes

Based on the above definitions, of these 135 patients 89 (65.9 per cent) were cured, 44 (32.6 per cent) got a fair or good effect and two (1.5 per cent) experienced no effect. Thus, overall, the effectiveness rate was 98.5 per cent.

Case history

The patient was a 21-year-old female. For five years she'd had nasal congestion, nasal itching and clear runny nose. Her symptoms were worse in the autumn and winter. However, she sometimes did have occurrences in the spring and summer. She was diagnosed as suffering from allergic rhinitis. She received moxibustion combined with the internal administration of Chinese medicinals. After five treatments, her nasal itching had disappeared, the flow of qi through both nostrils was free and fine and the runny nose had markedly diminished. She received a total of seven *ji* and two courses of moxibustion. After that, her symptoms completely disappeared and there was no recurrence on follow-up after one year.

Treatment Research 5

From 'The Treatment of 120 Cases of Allergic Rhinitis with *Suo Quan Wan Jia Jian* (Withdraw the Spring Pills with Additions and Subtractions)' by Chen De-jiang, *Yun Nan Zhong Yi Zhong Yao Za Zhi (Yunnan Journal of Chinese Medicine and Chinese Medicinals)*, No. 5, 1955

Suo Quan Wan is from the *Fu Ren Liang Fang* (Fine Formulae for Women). It is composed of Fructus Alpiniae Oxyphyllae *(Yi Zhi Ren)*, Radix Dioscoreae Oppositae *(Huai Shan Yao)* and Radix Linderae Strychnifoliae *(Wu Yao)*. Its function is to warm and strengthen the kidneys. It mainly treats deficiency and cold in the lower abdomen and kidneys leading to frequent urination and paediatric incontinence. Based on this clinical experience, the author has used this formula with modifications to treat 120 cases of allergic rhinitis with very good results.

Of these 120 patients, 50 were men and 70 were women. Their ages ranged from 17 to 45 years. The course of their disease had lasted from a minimum of one month to a maximum of four years. All these patients had been examined in the ear, nose and throat department.

Treatment method
The formula consisted of:

15 g/½ oz	Fructus Alpiniae Oxyphyllae *(Yi Zhi Ren)*
12 g/½ oz	Radix Dioscoreae Oppositae *(Shan Yao)*
10 g	Radix Linderae Strychnifoliae *(Wu Yao)*
15 g/½ oz	Radix Astragali Membranacei *(Huang Qi)*
10 g	Rhizoma Atractylodis *(Cang Zhu)*
10 g	Fructus Xanthii Sibirici *(Cang Er Zi)*
3 g,	Herba Cum Radice Asari Seiboldi *(Xi Xin)*
10 g	Flos Magnoliae Liliflorae *(Xin Yi)*
15 g/½ oz	Fructus Pruni Mume *(Wu Mei)*
15 g/½ oz	Fructus Schizandrae Chinensis *(Wu Wei Zi)*
6 g	Radix Ledebouriellae Divaricatae *(Fang Feng)*
3 g	Radix Glycyrrhizae *(Gan Cao)*

One *ji* was decocted and administered each day. A high fire was used and these medicinals were decocted twice. The first decoction was for 25 minutes and the second for 15 minutes. The two decoctions resulted in a combined volume of liquid of approximately 300 ml/½ pt. This was divided into two doses and administered on an empty stomach in the morning and evening.

Treatment outcomes
Of the 120 cases, after treatment the clinical symptoms disappeared and did not return within six months in 80 cases who were thus considered cured. In another 40 cases, the greater portion of their clinical symptoms disappeared.

However, they recurred within three months. In these cases, the protocol was considered to be markedly effective. Thus, overall, effectiveness rate was 100 per cent.

Discussion

Nei Jing (The Inner Classic) says, 'The lungs rule the mucus.' 'Difficulty 40' of *Nan Jing (Classic of Difficulties)* says, 'The lungs rule fluids.' Mucus is one of the five fluids and the five fluids are ruled by the kidneys. If the kidneys are vacuous, they do not store. Thus fluids and humours are discharged externally from the portal of the nose to become nasal mucus. Therefore, treatment should warm the kidneys and secure and astringe. This is why the author has chosen *Suo Quan Wan.* In addition, the lungs open into the portals of the nose. The lungs are the mother of the kidneys and it is said, 'If there is vacuity, supplement the mother.'

Thus it is appropriate to supplement the lungs and boost the qi, diffuse and free the flow of the portals of the nose. Hence the use of Alpinia, Dioscorea and Astragalus treats the root. Xanthium and Flos Magnoliae free the flow of the portals of the nose; Atractylodes and Asarum dry dampness, warm the lungs and transform rheum; while sour-flavoured Mume and Schizandra restrain, astringe and secure fluids and humours, thus treating the root. The lungs and kidneys are treated together, branch and root are simultaneously addressed and therefore a good effect is experienced.

CASE HISTORIES

In order to help readers get a better feel for how Chinese medicine treats respiratory allergies, I have included some more case histories. These are the stories of people who have benefited from treatment with Chinese medicine. It is my hope that these stories will encourage you to try acupuncture and Chinese medicine for yourself.

CASE 1

The patient was a 70-year-old retired woman. Her major complaint was allergic rhinitis and asthma from which she had suffered for over 60 years. When her allergies flared up in the spring and autumn or when she went near dogs and cats, itchy eyes and runny nose soon turned into asthmatic wheezing. If this continued for more than a day, she would then develop sinusitis. At the time of her first visit, the patient had a cough with copious white mucus. She had difficulty lying down and a tight chest. Clear, watery mucus flowed from her nose and her eyes were red and itchy.

In addition, she had heart palpitations, trouble going to sleep and was easily awoken during the night. She got up to urinate three to four times each night. Her hands and feet were cold, her ankles were slightly swollen with fluid and she caught cold easily. Her appetite and energy were both low, with two to three bowel movements per day. The stools themselves tended to be dry. She was currently being medicated with Prednisolone, Theodur (Theophylline), Proventrilo and Synthroid[5]. Her tongue was red with a deep

[5] Proventrilo and Synthroid are not available in the UK.

crack running down the centre with thick, white fur which was peeled in some areas. Her pulse was surging, slippery and rapid. Her Western medical diagnosis was allergic rhinitis and asthma with recurrent sinusitis.

Based on the above signs and symptoms, this woman's Chinese medical pattern discrimination was a (spleen) qi and (kidney) yin vacuity, with phlegm dampness obstructing her lungs. The treatment principles for this pattern are to fortify the spleen and supplement the qi, supplement the kidneys and enrich yin, transform phlegm, eliminate dampness and loosen the chest. Acupuncture treatment was given as follows:

Ying Xiang (Large intestine 20) for the runny nose
Zan Zhu (Bladder 2) for the itchy eyes
Tai Yuan (Lung 9) for the lungs
Tai Xi (Kidney 3) for the kidneys
San Yin Jiao (Spleen 6) for the spleen and kidneys
Zu San Li (Stomach 36) for the stomach and, therefore, the spleen
Feng Long (Stomach 40) for phlegm dampness
Shan Zhong (Conception vessel 17) to loosen the chest
Fei Shu (Bladder 13) for the lungs
Pi Shu (Bladder 20) for the spleen
Shen Shu (Bladder 23) for the kidneys

At the same time, she was prescribed two *ji* of Chinese herbs:

9 g Radix Pseudostellariae *(Tai Zi Shen)*
6 g Fructus Schisandrae Chinensis *(Wu Wei Zi)*
9 g Tuber Ophiopogonis Japonici *(Mai Men Dong)*
12 g Sclerotium Poriae Cocos *(Yun Fu Ling)*
9 g Rhizoma Dioscoreae Oppositae *(Huai Shan Yao)*
9 g Semen Pruni Armeniacae *(Ku Xing Ren)*
9 g Cortex Radicis Mori Albi *(Sang Bai Pi)*
9 g Folium Eriobotryae Japonicae *(Pi Pa Ye)*
6 g Semen Raphani Sativi *(Lai Fu Zi)*
6 g Mix-fried Radix Glycyrrhizae *(Zhi Gan Cao)*

In addition to the above Chinese herbs and acupuncture, the patient was advised to eat a clear, bland diet of cooked, not raw foods. In particular, she was instructed to stay away from sugars and sweets, dairy products (especially yoghurt and cheese), fruit juices, tomatoes and tomato sauce, peanuts and peanut butter and wheat as much as possible. She was asked particularly to stay away from yeasted bread. She was also taught how to do Chinese self-massage every day.

Two days later, the patient reported that her runny nose and itchy eyes had cleared up. She was surprised that her allergies had not developed into sinusitis. Her cough and the amount of phlegm in her lungs had decreased, but her chest was still tight and she still was able to cough up phlegm in the morning. Her energy was still low, but her appetite was better. Her tongue was red with peeled fur and her pulse was now bowstring and rapid. It was therefore decided to continue with basically the same Chinese herbal formula but to increase the ingredients for transforming phlegm and to add some ingredients for clearing heat from the liver. Thus the prescription now read:

9 g Folium Mori Albi *(Sang Ye)*
9 g Cortex Radicis Mori Albi *(Sang Bai Pi)*
9 g Flos Chrysanthemi Morifolii *(Ju Hua)*
9 g Tuber Ophiopogonis Japonici *(Mai Dong)*
9 g Radix Glehniae Littoralis *(Sha Shen)*
12 g Sclerotium Poriae Cocos *(Fu Ling)*
9 g Semen Pruni Armeniacae *(Xing Ren)*
9 g Bulbus Fritillariae Cirrhosae *(Chuan Bei Mu)*
9 g Pericarpium Trichosanthis Kirlowii *(Gua Lou Pi)*
6 g Radix Glycyrrhizae *(Gan Cao)*

The patient was given eight days' supply of this formula. At the same time, she received another acupuncture formula in order to boost her qi, transform phlegm and loosen her chest as well as clear heat from her liver. The acupuncture points consisted of:

Tai Chong (Liver 3) to course the liver and resolve depression
He Gu (Large intestine 4) to clear heat
Qu Chi (Large intestine 11) to clear heat
San Yin Jiao (Spleen 6) to supplement the spleen and kidneys
Lie Que (Lung 7) to diffuse the lungs
Zu San Li (Stomach 36) to supplement the spleen via the stomach
Shan Zhong (Conception vessel 17) to loosen the chest
Fei Shu (Bladder 13) for the lungs
Pi Shu (Bladder 20) for the spleen
Shen Shu (Bladder 23) for the kidneys

After one week, the patient reported that she was breathing much better. Her chest did not feel so tight, she was able to lie down and breathe easily and her energy was better. She was able to sleep better and she was only getting up once a night to urinate. She was adhering to the clear, bland diet quite well and she enjoyed doing the Chinese self-massage every day. As she was over the acute attack, she was taught how to do moxibustion in order to strengthen her spleen and kidneys. She was given several Chinese medicinal porridge recipes to include in her regular diet and a Chinese herbal prescription was written for more long-term root treatment.

This prescription was filled in the form of desiccated, powdered extracts which do not require cooking but are simply mixed with boiled water and drunk three times per day. The Chinese herbal prescription was called *Chang Shou Ba Wei Wan Jia Wei* (Long Life Eight Flavours Pills with Added Flavours). It consisted of:

12 g Tuber Ophiopogonis Japonici *(Mai Dong)*
9 g Fructus Schisandrae Chinensis *(Wu Wei Zi)*
12 g Cooked Radix Rehmanniae *(Shu Di)*
9 g Radix Dioscoreae Oppositae *(Shan Yao)*

9 g Fructus Cornus Officinalis *(Shan Zhu Yu)*
9 g Sclerotium Poriae Cocos *(Fu Ling)*
9 g Cortex Radicis Moutan *(Dan Pi)*
9 g Rhizoma Alismatis *(Ze Xie)*
9 g Bulbus Fritillariae Cirrhosae *(Chuan Bei Mu)*
9 g Radix Polygalae Tenuifoliae *(Yuan Zhi)*
15 g Mix-fried Radix Astragali Membranacei *(Huang Qi)*
9 g Cordyceps Sinensis *(Dong Chong Xia Cao)*

The woman continued on this formula for six months. On follow-up after one year, she had not had any allergic episodes and no asthma attacks. She was not getting up to urinate at night and she felt 10 years younger than her former self. Her doctor had taken her off all her Western medications except for the Synthroid.

CASE 2

The patient was a 10-year-old boy. He experienced bad hay fever each spring. When he went near cats, dogs, rabbits or horses he developed asthma. He also had a tendency to recurrent tonsillitis in the autumn and winter. His doctor had not suggested a tonsillectomy yet, but each winter the child was on antibiotics at least twice. He had been taking antibiotics off and on since he was seven months old when he had developed recurrent earaches. Currently, he had a copiously runny nose, sneezing and nasal congestion, red eyes, itchy eyes, throat and nose and pronounced irritability. The child was slightly overweight and the mother reported that he drank lots of orange juice, ate lots of ice cream, biscuits and chocolate and had a craving for bread. His tongue was swollen with the marks of his teeth on the borders of the tongue. The tongue fur was white and slightly slimy. His pulse was bowstring and slippery overall while being floating and fine in the right bar position (associated with the spleen) and floating and slippery in the right inch position (associated with the lungs).

This child's Chinese pattern discrimination was external invasion by wind evils with spleen vacuity, liver depression transforming heat and phlegm dampness. The treatment principles were to resolve the exterior and dispel wind, supplement the spleen and eliminate dampness, course and clear the liver and open the portals (of the nose). The boy didn't want needles so he was treated with a seven star hammer. This was tapped all along the back of his neck, his temples and all around the sides of his nose. In addition, *He Gu* (Large intestine 4) and *Tai Chong* (Liver 3) were tapped to resolve the exterior and course the liver, as was *Feng Long* (Stomach 40) in order to help transform phlegm. His mother then did seven star hammering every day for the next five days. At the same time, he was prescribed the following Chinese herbal formula:

9.0 g Radix Astragali Membranacei *(Huang Qi)*
4.5 g Radix Panacis Ginseng *(Ren Shen)*
6.0 g Rhizoma Atractylodis Macrocephalae *(Bai Zhu)*
6.0 g Rhizoma Pinelliae Ternatae *(Ban Xia)*
6.0 g Pericarpium Citri Reticulatae *(Chen Pi)*
9.0 g Sclerotium Poriae Cocos *(Fu Ling)*
4.5 g Mix-fried Radix Glycyrrhizae *(Gan Cao)*
3.0 g Radix Angelicae Sinensis *(Dang Gui)*
6.0 g Radix Schisandrae Chinensis *(Wu Wei Zi)*
1.5 g Herba Asari Cum Radice *(Xi Xin)*
6.0 g Radix Bupleuri *(Chai Hu)*
6.0 g Rhizoma Cimicifugae *(Sheng Ma)*
6.0 g Flos Chrysanthemi Morifolii *(Ju Hua)*
6.0 g Fructus Xanthii Sibirici *(Cang Er Zi)*
6.0 g Flos Magnoliae Liliflorae *(Xin Yi Hua)*

This prescription was administered for one week, at the end of which time the hay fever had disappeared. The child's mother was instructed on the clear, bland diet and she promised to do her best in getting her child to stick to this. This was in the spring and the child had no more hay fever that season. In the autumn, he was prescribed a modification of *Xiao Chai Hu Tang* (Minor Bupleurum Decoction) in desiccated, powdered extract form. This consisted of:

6.0 g Radix Bupleuri *(Chai Hu)*
4.5 g Radix Panacis Ginseng *(Ren Shen)*
6.0 g Radix Scutellariae Baicalensis *(Huang Qin)*
6.0 g Rhizoma Pinelliae Ternatae *(Ban Xia)*
6.0 g Pericarpium Citri Reticulatae *(Chen Pi)*
9.0 g Sclerotium Poriae Cocos *(Fu Ling)*
3.0 g Mix-fried Radix Glycyrrhizae *(Gan Cao)*
3 pieces Fructus Zizyphi Jujubae *(Da Zao)*
2 slices Uncooked Rhizoma Zingiberis *(Sheng Jiang)*

This was given from September to April. The child never caught a cold that year, did not have tonsillitis, did not have any hay fever in the spring and did not miss a single day of school that year.

According to Chinese medicine, antibiotics are excessively 'bitter and cold' and can damage the spleen. Although their use is sometimes warranted, they are often over- or unnecessarily prescribed. Although they do eliminate inflammation due to bacterial infection, they can also weaken the spleen. Since the spleen is the root of qi and blood production, including the defensive qi, damage of the spleen typically results in a defensive qi vacuity. This leaves the person open to easy attack as external wind evils take advantage of this vacuity to enter and cause disease. So it is not uncommon to see recurrent infections followed by repeated courses of antibiotics. The repeated antibiotics weaken the spleen. The person may be repeatedly invaded by wind evils. In such cases, it is extremely important to break this cycle by going without antibiotics unless absolutely necessary. As long as antibiotics are given again and again, the person's spleen has little chance of recuperating.

In addition, in this case we see that the child has a long history of complaints beginning in infancy. While these may be diagnosed as different diseases in Western medicine, from a Chinese medical point of view these are seen as a continuum, certain diseases occurring at certain ages, but all due to spleen vacuity with accumulation of phlegm and dampness. For more information on Chinese medicine and children's diseases, read *Keeping Your Child Healthy with Chinese Medicine* (see page 154).

CASE 3

The patient was a 43-year-old female airline pilot. She said her hormones were 'on a rampage' and that she was having allergic reactions to many things. When asked what these things were, she said dogs and cats. She had been allergic to these younger in her life but then had 'outgrown' the problem. Now it was coming back, with coughing and red, painful, itchy eyes. The cough was dry, occasionally there was wheezing and her chest felt tight. On her inner arms she had a skin rash that had previously been made up of many small blisters. Now it was a diffuse red rash which was very itchy. Her menstruation had come recently four days late instead of several days early. She complained that her eyes were always irritated and out of focus. She had continuous headaches right behind her eyes and occasionally in the middle of the back of her head. Her memory was 'off' and her focus was not good. Her bowel movements were fine, but her appetite had lessened. Nonetheless, she had gained about 3 kg/6 lb in the last year. Her energy levels were good in the morning but then 'crashed' at 3 p.m. and she was in bed by 9 p.m. She slept 'like a log'. In addition, she had severe lower back pain, her feet were always cold and she had zero libido.

The patient's tongue was light red, swollen, had the marks of her teeth on its edges, was darker all around its rim and had thin, white fur. Her pulse was floating and slippery in the right inch position (associated with the lungs), bowstring and floating in the right bar (associated with the spleen) and fine, bowstring and not very forceful in the right cubit (associated with kidney yang). On the left, the inch (associated with the heart) was floating vacuous, the bar (associated with the liver) was bowstring and the cubit (associated with kidney yin) was fine, a little bowstring and less forceful than the right cubit.

All this adds up to the following Chinese pattern discrimination: depressive heat in the liver and lungs damaging fluids, spleen vacuity and kidney yang vacuity. The treatment principles were to resolve depression, clear the liver and lungs, fortify the spleen, boost the qi, invigorate the kidneys and strengthen the lower back. In addition, because it was day 17 in her menstrual cycle, the principles of quickening the blood and regulating menstruation were also used. Since the woman lived 2,000 miles away, a formula was written but no acupuncture was given. The formula consisted of:

9 g	Radix Bupleuri *(Chai Hu)*
18 g	Radix Astragali Membranacei *(Huang Qi)*
9 g	Radix Codonopsitis Pilosulae *(Dang Shen)*
9 g	Radix Dioscoreae Oppositae *(Shan Yao)*
9 g	Sclerotium Poriae Cocos *(Fu Ling)*
12 g	Tuber Ophiopogonis Japonici *(Mai Dong)*
12 g	Radix Scutellariae Baicalensis *(Huang Qin)*
9 g	Fructus Gardeniae Jasminoidis *(Shan Zhi Zi)*
9 g	Flos Chrysanthemi Morifolii *(Ju Hua)*
9 g	Radix Rubrus Paeoniae Lactiflorae *(Chi Shao)*
15 g	Radix Ligustici Wallichii *(Chuan Xiong)*
9 g	Radix Angelicae Sinensis *(Dang Gui)*

12 g Uncooked Radix Rehmanniae *(Sheng Di)*
9 g Cortex Eucommiae Ulmoidis *(Du Zhong)*
9 g Radix Dipsaci *(Xu Duan)*
6 g Mix-fried Radix Glycyrrhizae *(Gan Cao)*
3 pieces Fructus Zizyphi Jujubae *(Da Zao)*
3 slices Uncooked Rhizoma Zingiberis *(Sheng Jiang)*

This formula was prescribed for three days. At the end of this time, the patient called to say that the headaches were gone, her eyes were slightly clearer and her skin had no red bumps. However, her skin still itched. Therefore, her formula was rewritten to include 15 g Fructus Tribuli Terrestris *(Bai Ji Li)*, for the itching, while the red dates and ginger were subtracted as being essentially superfluous.

After 10 days, the patient called in again. Now she said that everything was definitely better. Her menstruation had come on time and the blood was much less clotted. Her lower back pain was better. However, her skin still itched and she had lots of wind each time she drank the herbs. Therefore, her prescription was again rewritten in order to make it more effective without any side-effects:

18 g Radix Astragali Membranacei *(Huang Qi)*
12 g Cooked Radix Rehmanniae *(Shu Di)*
9 g Radix Angelicae Sinensis *(Dang Gui)*
15 g Radix Dioscoreae Oppositae *(Shan Yao)*
9 g Fructus Corni Officinalis *(Shan Zhu Yu)*
9 g Sclerotium Poriae Cocos *(Fu Ling)*
9 g Cortex Radicis Moutan *(Dan Pi)*
9 g Flos Chrysanthemi Morifollii *(Ju Hua)*
9 g Radix Scutellariae Baicalensis *(Huang Qin)*
12 g Tuber Ophiopogonis Japonici *(Mai Dong)*
15 g Fructus Tribuli Terrestris *(Bai Ji Li)*
9 g Bombyx Batryticatus *(Jiang Can)*
9 g Radix Ledebouriellae Divaricatae *(Fang Feng)*
9 g Herba Seu Flos Schizonepetae Tenuifoliae *(Jing Jie)*

These modifications were meant to reduce the abdominal bloating and at the same time more effectively eliminate the skin itching. At the end of another two weeks, the patient reported that all her symptoms had been eliminated and that she felt great!

FINDING A PROFESSIONAL PRACTITIONER OF CHINESE MEDICINE

Chinese medicine has grown enormously in the UK during the past 30 years. There are at least ten colleges which offer a professional training, some offering a university degree. Many excellent practitioners have come to the UK from China, Vietnam and other countries of East Asia.

As you will no doubt have realised after reading this book, Chinese medicine is a whole system of medicine with its own fundamental concepts and theories. It is not simply a technique. Previous knowledge or training in another system of medicine does not automatically confer competence or knowledge in Chinese medicine. In order to get the most out of your therapy or treatment you should ensure that the practitioner is properly qualified. Currently in the UK the onus is on the public to check the qualifications and training of their practitioner. In order to help you to do this I have listed the relevant professional bodies covering Chinese medicine. Members of these professional organisations are bound by a professional code of ethics and practice. They will have received an accredited level of training and will be covered by medical malpractice and public/products liability insurance.

When trying to find a good practitioner, one of the best methods is personal recommendation. It is also important that you are able to communicate with the practitioner should English not be their first language. It is quite acceptable to ask about their previous experience in treating your complaint. Many practitioners will be happy to talk on the phone or may offer a short introductory consultation so that you can assess whether you will feel comfortable working with them.

I have included Japanese traditions of herbal medicine (kanpo) and massage (shiatsu) in addition to Chinese. They originate from the same basic sources but have evolved differently in terms of style and practice.

The relevant professional bodies in the UK are:

Acupuncture
The British Acupuncture Council
63 Jeddo Road
London
W12 9HQ
Tel: 020 8735 0400
Fax: 020 8735 0404
E-mail: infor@acupuncture.org.uk
Website: www.acupuncture.org.uk

Members have the initials: MBAcC.

Chinese herbal medicine
The Register of Chinese Herbal Medicine
PO Box 400
Wembley
Middlesex
HA9 9NZ
Tel/fax: 07000 790332
Website: www.rchm.co.uk

Members have the initials: MRCHM.

Japanese herbal medicine
The Kanpo Association
9a Ingatestone Road
Brentwood
Essex
CM15 8AP
Tel: 01277 260080

Members have the initials: KANPO.
Members of the Kanpo Association are not bound by a code of ethics and practice or covered by insurance unless they also belong to another professional body. Most practitioners of kanpo belong to one of the three other professional bodies.

Shiatsu
The Shiatsu Society UK
Barber House
Storeys Bar Road
Fengate
Peterborough
PE1 5YS
Tel: 01733 758341
E-mail: shiatsu@graphic-scan.co.uk

Members have the initials: MRSS.

Relevant bodies in other English-speaking countries are:

Australian Acupuncture & Chinese Medical Association (AACMA)
PO Box 5142
West End
Brisbane
Queensland
Australia 4101
Tel: +07 3846 5866
Fax: +07 3846 5276
Free Call: 1800 025 334
E-mail: aaca@eis.net.all
Website: http://www2.eis.net.au/-aaca

The International Institute of Chinese Medicine and Acupuncture
PO Box 2246
19 Av Disandt-Fresnaye
Cape Town 8000
South Africa
Tel: 27 21 434 1654

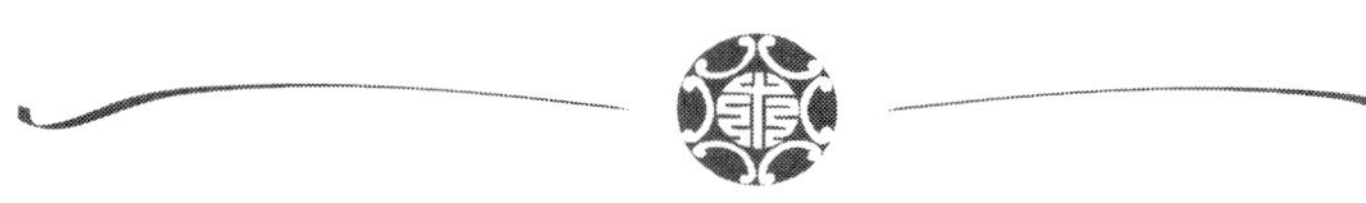

LEARNING MORE ABOUT CHINESE MEDICINE

Chinese medicine in general

Chinese Medicine: Acupuncture, Herbal Remedies, Nutrition, Qui Gong and Meditation, Tom Williams, Element Health Essentials
This is a good basic introduction to the whole field of Chinese medicine for the layperson.

Acupuncture, Peter Mole, Element Books
A simple and clear introduction to acupuncture for the layperson.

A Guide to Acupuncture, Peter Firebrace and Sandra Hill, Constable Books
A comprehensive introduction to acupuncture for the layperson with some illustrations and photographs.

Between Heaven and Earth: A Guide to Chinese Medicine, Harriet Beinfield and Efrem Corngold, Ballantine Books, New York
This book is particularly good with regard to the more psychological and emotional aspects of Chinese medicine and has a good introduction to herbal medicine for the layperson.

Acupuncture in Practice, Hugh McPherson and Ted Kaptchuk (eds), Churchill Livingston
This is a book of case histories from the West; it illustrates the wide variety of styles and methods of practice of acupuncture by many well-known practitioners.

Chinese Herbal Medicine, a Practical Guide to the Healing Powers of Herbs, Dr Guang Xu, Vermillion
A good introduction to Chinese herbal medicine.

Japanese Acupuncture, a Clinical Guide, Stephen Birch and Junko Ida, Paradigm Publications
This book gives very good, clear instructions on moxibustion.

Chinese dietary therapy

Healing with Wholefoods, Oriental Traditions and Modern Nutrition, Paul Pritchard, North Atlantic Books
A comprehensive source book for both the layperson and the professional.

Helping Ourselves: A Guide to the Traditional Chinese Food Energetics, Daverick Legget, Meridian Press
This book is designed for ease of use with its clear layout and wallcharts.

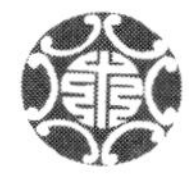

SUPPLIERS OF CHINESE MEDICINES

Acumedic
101–5 Camden High Street
London
NW1 7JN
Tel: 0171 388 5783
Fax: 0171 387 5766

Beijing Tong Ren Tang
124 Shaftesbury Avenue
London
W1V 7DJ
Tel: 0171 287 0098
Fax: 0171 287 0068

China Medica
25 Lonsdale Close
London
SE9 4HF
Tel: 0181 857 9777
Fax: 0181 480 2020

Chinese Medical Centre
179 South Street
Romford
Essex
RM1 1PS
Tel: 01708 756363
Fax: 01708 703015

East West Herbs
Langston Priory Mews
Kingham
Oxfordshire
OX7 6UP
Tel: 01608 658862
Fax: 01608 658816
E-mail: robert@eastwestherbs.co.uk

Great Wall
Unit 27
Riverside Works
Hertford Road
Barking
Essex
IG11 8BN
Tel: 0181 591 6896
Fax: 0181 591 6891

Harmony Medical Distribution
629 High Road
Leytonstone
London
E11 4PA
Tel: 0181 518 7337
Fax: 0181 556 5038
E-mail: harmony@tcm.org.uk

Lotus
Priorsfield Priory
Forest Row
Sussex
RH18 5HR
Tel: 01342 823053
Fax: 01342 826027
E-mail: user@lotus.u-net.com

Mayway UK
43 Waterside Trading Centre
Trumpers Way
Hanwell
Middlesex
Tel: 0181 893 6873
Fax: 0181 893 6874

Naturally Chinese
P.O. Box 4584
Kiln Farm
Milton Keynes
Bucks
MK13 9BT
Tel: 0151 571 0407

Number One Herb Co.
36 Bankhurst Road
Catford
London
SE6 4XN
Tel: 0181 690 4840
Fax: 0181 690 4840
E-mail: jarrah@vossnet.co.uk

Oxford Medical Supplies
Units 11 & 12
Horcott Industrial Estate
Fairford
Gloucestershire
GL7 4LX
Tel: 0800 975 8000
Fax: 0800 975 8111
E-mail: oxfordms@demon.co.uk

Shizhen TCM UK Ltd
50 Sandy Lane
Chorlton
Manchester
M21
Tel: 0161 881 0088
Fax: 0161 881 0888

Tian Tiao Ltd
85 Sullivan Way
Elstree
Herts
WD6 3DG
Tel: 0181 953 2320
Fax: 0181 953 3338

CHINESE MEDICAL GLOSSARY

Chinese medicine is a system unto itself. Its technical terms are uniquely its own and cannot be reduced to the definitions of Western medicine without destroying the very fabric and logic of Chinese medicine. Ultimately, because Chinese medicine was created in the Chinese language, Chinese medicine is best and really only understood in that language. Nevertheless, as Westerners trying to understand Chinese medicine, we must translate the technical terms of Chinese medicine into English words. If some of these technical translations sound at first peculiar and their meaning is not immediately clear, this is because no equivalent concepts exist in everyday English.

In the past, some Western authors have erroneously translated technical Chinese medical terms using Western medical or at least quasi-scientific words in an attempt to make this system more acceptable to Western audiences. For instance, the words tonify and sedate are commonly seen in the Western Chinese medical literature even though, in the case of sedate, its meaning is completely opposite to the Chinese understanding of the word *xie*. *Xie* means to drain off something that has pooled and accumulated. That accumulation is seen as something excess which should not be lingering where it is. Because it is accumulating somewhere where it shouldn't, it is impeding and obstructing whatever should be moving into and through that area. The word sedate comes from the Latin word *sedere*, to sit. Therefore, the word sedate means to make something sit still. In English, we get the word sediment from this same root. However, the Chinese *xie* means draining off that which is sitting somewhere erroneously.

Therefore, to think that one is going to sedate what is already sitting is a great mistake in understanding the clinical implication and application of this technical term.

Hence, in order to preserve the integrity of this system while still making it intelligible to English language readers, I have appended the following glossary of Chinese medical technical terms. The terms themselves are based on Nigel Wiseman's *English–Chinese Chinese–English Dictionary of Chinese Medicine* (see Bibliography, page 153). Dr Wiseman is, I believe, the greatest Western scholar in terms of the translation of Chinese medicine into English. As a Chinese reader myself, although I often think Wiseman's terms sound awkward at first, I also think they convey most accurately the Chinese understanding and logic of these terms.

Acquired essence: Essence manufactured out of the surplus of qi and blood in turn created out of the refined essence of food and drink

Acupoints: Those places on the channels and network vessels where qi and blood tend to collect in denser concentrations and thus those places where the qi and blood in the channels are especially available for manipulation

Acupuncture: The regulation of qi flow by the stimulation of certain points located on the channels and network vessels achieved mainly by insertion of fine needles into these points

Bar: A position on the radial artery of the wrist, where the pulse is felt

Bedroom taxation: Fatigue or vacuity due to excessive sex

Blood: The red-coloured fluids that flow in the vessels and nourish and construct the tissues of the body

Blood stasis: Also called dead blood, malign blood and dry blood, blood stasis is blood that is no longer moving through the vessels as it should. Instead it is precipitated in the vessels like silt in a river. It obstructs the free flow of the blood in the vessels and also impedes the production of new or fresh blood

Blood vacuity: Insufficient blood manifesting in diminished nourishment, construction and moistening of body tissues

Bowels: The hollow yang organs of Chinese medicine

Bowstring pulse: A pulse that feels like a tight, taut string

Burner: One of the three areas of the abdomen, known respectively as the upper, middle and lower burners, that act as a kind of crucible within which the vital energies are transformed and created by heat

Central qi: Also called the middle qi, this is synonymous with the spleen-stomach qi

Channels: The main routes for the distribution of blood and, in particular, qi

Clear: The pure or clear part of food and drink ingested which is then turned into qi and blood

Cold: A pathogenic factor that can invade the body from the outside environment. May combine with wind to form wind cold invasion. Can also be produced as a weakness of internal physiological processes. Cold may be 'scattered', i.e. broken up and released from the body through treatment

Constructive qi: The qi that flows through the channels and nourishes and constructs the internal organs and body tissues

Counterflow: An erroneous flow of qi, usually upwards but sometimes horizontally as well

Course the liver: Encourage the correct functioning of the liver viscera with regard to the flow of qi throughout the body

Cubit body: A position on the radial artery of the wrist where the pulse is felt

Damp heat: A combination of accumulated dampness mixed with pathological heat often associated with sores, abnormal vaginal discharges and some types of menstrual and body pain

Dampness: A pathological accumulation of body fluids

Decoction: A method of administering Chinese medicinals by boiling these medicinals in water, removing the dregs and drinking the resulting medicinal liquid

Defensive qi: The yang qi that protects the exterior of the body from invasion by the environmental excesses

Depression: Stagnation and lack of movement, as in liver depression qi stagnation

Depressive heat: Heat due to enduring or severe qi stagnation, which then transforms into heat

Drain: To drain off or away some pathological qi or substance from where it is replete (excessive)

Environmental excesses: A superabundance of wind, cold, dampness, dryness, heat or summer heat in the external environment, which can invade the body and cause disease

Essence: A stored, very potent form of substance and qi, usually yin when compared to yang qi, but can be transformed into yang qi

External causes of disease: The six environmental excesses (see above)

Fire: A pathogenic factor that is usually created within the body. In addition, initial invasion by an external pathogenic factor, such as wind cold, may transform into fire within the body

Fine pulse: A pulse that feels delicate

Five-phase theory: An ancient Chinese system of correspondences dividing up all of reality into five phases, which then mutually engender and check each other according to definite sequences

Floating pulse: A pulse that can be felt on a superficial level, with a 'floating' quality

Heat: A pathogenic factor, usually external, i.e. from the environment

Heat toxins: A particularly virulent and concentrated type of pathological heat often associated with purulence (i.e. pus formation), sores and sometimes, but not always, malignancies

Impediment: A hindrance to the free flow of the qi and blood typically manifesting as pain and restriction in the range of movement of a joint or extremity

Inch: A position on the radial artery of the wrist where the pulse is felt

Internal causes of disease: The seven effects or emotions, namely, anger, joy (or excitement), sorrow, thought, fear, melancholy and fright

Lassitude of the spirit: A listless or apathetic effect or emotional demeanour due to obvious fatigue of the mind and body

Life gate fire: Another name for kidney yang or kidney fire, seen as the ultimate source of yang qi in the body

Mansion: Realm of influence of one of the viscera

Middle burner *see* **Burner**

Moxibustion: Burning the herb *Artemisia Argyium* on, over or near acupuncture points in order to add yang qi, to warm cold, or promote the movement of the qi and blood

Neither external nor internal causes of disease: A miscellaneous group of pathogenic factors including trauma, diet, overwork, insufficient exercise, poisoning and parasites

Network vessels: Small vessels which form a net-like web ensuring the flow of qi and blood to all body tissues

Pattern discrimination: Basis for diagnosis in TCM. A pattern is determined based on signs and symptoms and observations of the individual patient's condition

Phlegm: A pathological accumulation of phlegm or mucus congealed from dampness or body fluids

Portals: Also called orifices, the openings of the sensory organs (e.g. the nostrils, ears, etc.) and the opening of the heart through which the spirit makes contact with the world outside

Qi: Activity, function, that which moves, transforms, defends, restrains and warms

Qi mechanism: The process of transforming yin substance controlled and promoted by the qi, largely synonymous with the process of digestion

Qi vacuity: Insufficient qi manifesting in diminished movement, transformation and function

Repletion: Excess or fullness, almost always pathological

Resolve the exterior: Release and clear the pathogens from the outer layers of the body, where its primary defence mechanisms are located

Root: Refers to an underlying pattern of illness, as opposed to more superficial or temporary disorders

Scatter *see* **Cold**

Seven star hammer: A small hammer with needles embedded in its head, used to stimulate acupoints without actually inserting needles

Slippery pulse: A pulse quality that often denotes the presence of phlegm or dampness in the body

Spirit: The accumulation of qi in the heart, which manifests as consciousness, sensory awareness and mental-emotional function

Stagnation: Non-movement of the qi, lack of free flow, constraint

Supplement: To add to or augment, as in supplementing the qi, blood, yin, or yang

Turbid: The yin, impure, turbid part of food and drink, which is sent downwards to be excreted as waste

Vacuity: Emptiness or insufficiency, typically of qi, blood, yin, or yang

Vacuity cold: Obvious signs and symptoms of cold due to a lack or insufficiency of yang qi

Vacuity heat: Heat due to hyperactive yang, in turn due to insufficient controlling yin

Vessels: The main routes for the distribution of qi and blood, but mainly blood

Viscera: The solid yin organs of Chinese medicine

Wind cold invasion: When the external pathogens of wind and cold have broken through the body's defences

Wind evils: External pathogenic factors, unseen pathogens that invade the body's defences

Yang: In the body, function, movement, activity, transformation

Yang vacuity: Insufficient warming and transforming function giving rise to symptoms of cold in the body

Yin: In the body, substance and nourishment

Yin vacuity: Insufficient yin substance necessary to nourish, control and counterbalance yang activity

BIBLIOGRAPHY

CHINESE LANGUAGE SOURCES

Shang Hai Lao Zhong Yi Jing Yan Xuan Bian (A Selected Compilation of Shanghai Old Doctors' Experiences). Shanghai Science and Technology Press, Shanghai, 1984.

Hou Tian-yin and Wang Chun-hua, *Tan Zheng Lun (Treatise on Phlegm Conditions).* People's Army Press, Beijing, 1989.

Hu Zhao-ming (ed.), *Zhong Guo Zhong Yi Mi Fang Da Quan (A Great Compendium of Chinese National Medical Secret Formulas).* Literary Propagation Publishing Company, Shanghai, 1992.

Huang Xiao-kai, *Han Ying Chang Yong Yi Xue Ci Hui (Chinese–English Glossary of Commonly Used Medical Terms).* People's Health and Hygiene Press, Beijing, 1982.

Li Shou-xian, *Zhen Jiu Yi Xue (An Easy Study of Acupuncture and Moxibustion).* People's Health and Hygiene Press, Beijing, 1990.

Li Zhong-yu, *Chu Zhen Zhi Liao Xue (A Study of Acupuncture Treatment).* Sichuan Science and Technology Press, Chengdu, 1990.

Lin Bin-zhi, *Zhong Yi Ling Yan Fang (Efficacious Chinese Medical Formulas).* Science and Technology Propagation Press, Beijing, 1991.

Liu Guang-rui and Liu Shao-lin, *Zhong Guo Min Jian Cao Yao Fang (Chinese Folk Herbal Medicinal Formulas)*. Sichuan Science and Technology Press, Chengdu, 1992.

Lu Su-ying, *Zhong Yi Hu Li Xue (A Study of Chinese Medical Nursing)*. People's Health and Hygiene Press, Beijing, 1983.

Qiu Mao-liang *et al.*, *Zhen Jiu Xue (A Study of Acupuncture and Moxibustion)*. Shanghai Science and Technology Press, Shanghai, 1985.

Wu Qian *et al.*, *Yi Zong Jin Jian (The Golden Mirror of Ancestral Medicine)*. People's Health and Hygiene Press, Beijing, 1985.

Xia Zhi-ping, *Shi Yong Zhen Jiu Tui Na Zhi Liao Xue (A Study of Practical Acupuncture, Moxibustion and Tui Na Treatments)*. Shanghai College of Chinese Medicine Press, Shanghai, 1990.

Xiao Shao-qing, *Zhong Guo Zhen Jiu Chu Fang Xue (A Study of Chinese Acupuncture and Moxibustion Prescriptions)*. Ningxia People's Press, Yinchuan, 1986.

Yang Ji-zhou, *Zhen Jiu Da Cheng (A Great Compendium of Acupuncture and Moxibustion)*. People's Health and Hygiene Press, Beijing, 1983.

Zhang En-qin *et al.*, *Zhong Yi Lin Chuang Ge Ke (Various Clinical Specialties in Chinese Medicine)*. Shanghai College of TCM Press, Shanghai, 1990.

Zhang En-qin (ed.), *A Practical English–Chinese Library of Traditional Chinese Medicine (II)*. Shanghai College of Traditional Chinese Medicine Publishing House, Shanghia, 1990.

ENGLISH LANGUAGE SOURCES

A Barefoot Doctor's Manual, revised and enlarged edition, Cloud Burst Press, Mayne Isle, 1977.

Bensky, Dan and Barolet, Randall *Chinese Herbal Medicine: Formulas and Strategies.* Eastland Press, Seattle, 1990.

Bensky, Dan and Gamble, Andrew *Chinese Herbal Medicine: Materia Medica* (second revised edition). Eastland Press, Seattle, 1993.

Berkow, Robert (ed.), *The Merck Manual,* 15th edition. Merck Sharp and Dohme Research Laboratories, Rahway, New Jersey, 1987.

Chen Ze-lin and Chen Mei-fang, *A Comprehensive Guide to Chinese Herbal Medicine.* Oriental Healing Arts Institute, Long Beach, California, 1992.

Cheng Song-yu and Li Fei, *A Clinical Guide to Chinese Herbs and Formulae.* Churchill and Livingstone, Edinburgh, 1993.

Eckman, Peter *In the Footsteps of the Yellow Emperor: Tracing the History of Traditional Acupuncture.* Cypress Book Co., San Francisco, 1996.

Ellis, Andrew; Wiseman, Nigel and Boss, Ken *Fundamentals of Chinese Acupuncture.* Paradigm Publications, Brookline, Massachusetts, 1988.

Fan Ya-li, *Chinese Self-massage Therapy, The Easy Way to Health.* Blue Poppy Press, Boulder, Colorado, 1996.

Farquhar, Judith *Knowing Practice: The Clinical Encounter of Chinese Medicine.* Westview Press, Boulder, Colorado, 1994.

Flaws, Bob and Finney, Daniel *A Compendium of TCM Patterns and Treatments.* Blue Poppy Press, Boulder, Colorado, 1996.

Flaws, Bob *The Dao of Healthy Eating According to Traditional Chinese Medicine.* Blue Poppy Press, Boulder, Colorado, 1997.

Flaws, Bob *Keeping Your Child Healthy with Chinese Medicine.* Blue Poppy Press, Boulder, Colorado.

Flaws, Bob *Chinese Medicinal Wines and Elixirs.* Blue Poppy Press, Boulder, Colorado, 1995.

Flaws, Bob *Statements of Fact in Traditional Chinese Medicine.* Blue Poppy Press, Boulder, Colorado, 1994.

Flaws, Bob *The Book of Jook: Chinese Medicinal Porridges.* Blue Poppy Press, Boulder, Colorado, 1995.

Geng Jun-ying, *et al., Practical Traditional Chinese Medicine and Pharmacology: Herbal Formulas.* New World Press, Beijing, 1991.

Him-che Yeung, *Handbook of Chinese Herbs and Formulas.* Self-published, Los Angeles, 1985.

Hong-yen Hsu, *Oriental Materia Medica, A Concise Guide.* Oriental Healing Arts Institute, Long Beach, California, 1986.

Li Dong-yuan, (trans. Yang Shou-zhong), *The Treatise on the Spleen and Stomach.* Blue Poppy Press, Boulder, Colorado, 1993.

Liu Yan-chi, (trans. Fang Ting-yu and Chen Lai-di), *The Essential Book of Traditional Chinese Medicine.* Columbia University Press, New York, 1988.

Ou Ming (ed.), *Chinese–English Manual of Common-used Prescriptions in Traditional Chinese Medicine.* Joint Publishing Co. Ltd, Hong Kong, 1989.

Ou-yang Yi, (trans. C.S. Cheung), *A Handbook of Differential Diagnosis with Key Signs and Symptoms, Therapeutic Principles and Guiding Prescriptions.* Harmonious Sunshine Cultural Centre, San Francisco, 1987.

Reid, Daniel *The Complete Book of Chinese Health and Healing.* Shambhala, Boston, Massachusetts, 1994.

Ross, Jeremy *Zang Fu: The Organ Systems of Traditional Chinese Medicine* (second edition). Churchill Livingstone, Edinburgh, 1985.

Shang Xian-min *et al., Practical Traditional Chinese Medicine and Pharmacology: Clinical Experiences.* New World Press, Beijing, 1990.

Shuai Xue-zhong *et al., Chinese–English Terminology of Traditional Chinese Medicine.* Hunan Science and Technology Press, Changsha, 1983.

Sivin, Nathan *Traditional Medicine in Contemporary China.* University of Michigan, Ann Arbor, 1987.

Unschuld, Paul U. *Medicine in China: A History of Ideas.* University of California Press, Berkeley, 1985.

Wiseman, Nigel *English–Chinese Chinese–English Dictionary of Chinese Medicine*. Hunan Science and Technology Press, Changsha, 1995.

Wiseman, Nigel and Boss, Ken *A Glossary of Chinese Medical Terms and Acupuncture Points*. Paradigm Publications, Brookline, Massachusetts, 1990.

Wiseman, Nigel and Ellis, Andrew *Fundamentals of Chinese Medicine*. Paradigm Publications, Brookline, Massachusetts, 1985.

Xuan Jia-sheng (ed.), *The English–Chinese Encyclopedia of Practical Traditional Chinese Medicine*. Higher Education Press, Beijing, 1990.

Zong Xiao-fan and Gary Liscum, *Chinese Medicinal Teas: Simple, Proven Folk Formulas for the Treatment of Disease and Promotion of Health*. Blue Poppy Press, Boulder, Colorado, 1997.

INDEX